THE
LEAN
LOOK

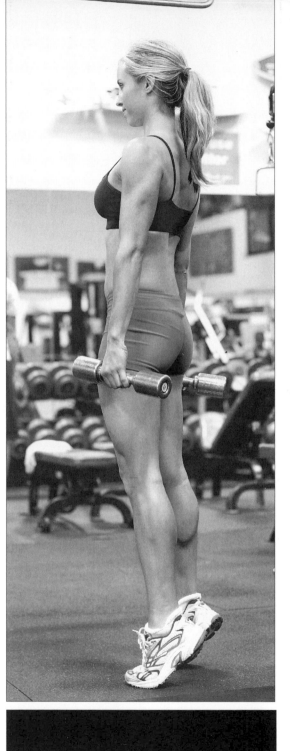

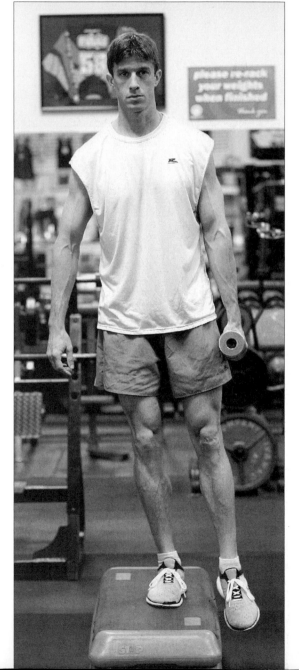

THE
LEAN
LOOK

Burn Fat, Tone Muscles, and Transform Your Body in Twelve Weeks Using the Secrets of Professional Athletes

Paul Goldberg
and
Matt Fitzgerald

BROADWAY BOOKS
New York

BROADWAY

PUBLISHED BY BROADWAY BOOKS

Copyright © 2008 by Matthew Fitzgerald and Paul Goldberg

All Rights Reserved

Published in the United States by Broadway Books, an imprint of The Doubleday Broadway Publishing Group, a division of Random House, Inc., New York.

www.broadwaybooks.com

BROADWAY BOOKS and its logo, a letter B bisected on the diagonal, are trademarks of Random House, Inc.

Healthy Body Fat Percentage Ranges table adapted with permission from the *American Journal of Clinical Nutrition* (2000; vol. 72; 694–701), American Society for Nutrition.

Book design by Nicola Ferguson

Library of Congress Cataloging-in-Publication Data

Goldberg, Paul, 1967–
The lean look : burn fat, tone muscles, and transform your body in twelve weeks using the secrets of professional athletes / Paul Goldberg and Matt Fitzgerald. — 1st ed.
p. cm.
1. Weight training. 2. Cardiovascular fitness. 3. Nutrition. I. Fitzgerald, Matt. II. Title.
GV546.G65 2007
613.7'12—dc22   2007028762

ISBN 978-0-7679-2589-1

PRINTED IN THE UNITED STATES OF AMERICA

10 9 8 7 6 5 4 3 2 1

First Edition

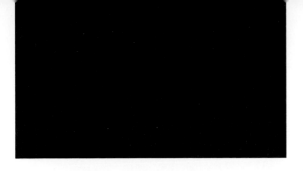

CONTENTS

INTRODUCTION: Meet the Dean of Lean, *1*

CHAPTER 1: Why Leaner Is Better, *7*

CHAPTER 2: How to Measure Your Leanness, *14*

CHAPTER 3: An Overview of the Lean Look Program, *20*

PHASE I

CHAPTER 4: Introduction to Phase I, *33*

CHAPTER 5: Nutrition: Key Food Substitutions, *38*

CHAPTER 6: Resistance Exercise: Muscle Balancing, *59*

CHAPTER 7: Cardio Exercise: Short Intervals, *98*

PHASE II

CHAPTER 8: Introduction to Phase II, *121*

CHAPTER 9: Nutrition: Nutrient Timing, *126*

CHAPTER 10: Resistance Exercise: Strength Building, *145*

CHAPTER 11: Cardio Exercise: Intermediate Intervals, *185*

PHASE III

CHAPTER 12: Introduction to Phase III, *197*

CHAPTER 13: Nutrition: Smart Supplementation, *202*

CHAPTER 14: Resistance Exercise: Power Development, *219*

CHAPTER 15: Cardio Exercise: Long Intervals, *245*

CHAPTER 16: Lean for Life, *258*

APPENDIX A: Body Fat Estimation Tables for Use with the Tape Measure Method, *267*

APPENDIX B: A Sample Four-Week Lean Look Meal Plan, *278*

APPENDIX C: Resources, *283*

INDEX *289*

THE
LEAN
LOOK

INTRODUCTION

Meet the Dean
of Lean

A lot of men and women come to my fitness facility in hopes that I can help them lose weight. But I don't help anyone lose weight. I help them do something much better: get lean. The method that is most effective for losing weight—crash dieting—is different from the most effective methods for getting lean, which you'll learn about in this book.

Turns out, your weight is not important. The bathroom scale tells you very little about your health, your fitness, or even your appearance. What does matter is your *body composition*, or the relative proportions of fat tissue and fat-free tissue (mainly muscle) in your body. The most common way of assessing body composition is by measuring body fat percentage. A low body fat percentage is ideal. However, having a low body fat percentage is different from having a low body weight. If you're tall, large-framed, or muscular, you could have a high body weight but have a low body fat percentage. On the other hand, you could have a low body weight and even look "skinny" yet still have a high body fat percentage—a phenomenon called *normal weight obesity.*

Health scientists and medical doctors used to believe that body weight was important. But within the past decade a revolution has occurred: The latest research has clearly shown that body composition is a much better indicator of overall health than body weight. Lowering one's body fat percentage is proven to reduce the risk of heart disease, diabetes, various cancers, Alzheimer's disease, and other ailments. It also improves energy levels, work performance, confidence, mood, and stress levels. What's more, psychological research shows that a low body fat physique is also the most attractive physique for both sexes. Men prefer lean women to skinny women, and women prefer lean men to both skinny and overly muscular men. And now you can enjoy these benefits of leanness by following the simple and effective 12-week Lean Look program presented in this book.

Most of my clients are skeptical when I first steer them away from the medical scale toward the BOD POD—a high-tech device in my facility that measures body fat percentage with a high degree of accuracy. But in the end they are always glad I did. With my clients I push the message that leanness is more important than weight so much that one of them nicknamed me "The Dean of Lean"—and it stuck!

My journey toward becoming the Dean of Lean began in a small city just north of San Diego called Escondido—a virtual paradise for the sort of active kid I was. My family had orange groves, as did all the families on our street, and every day the neighborhood kids and I ran and played in them from dawn to dusk. There was no such thing as Game Boy, so we rode our bikes everywhere and passed the time with outdoor games instead. From these early experiences I learned that exercise can and should be fun.

In my early teens I discovered that I was stronger than most kids and I became interested in weight lifting. Luckily we had a terrific strength coach in our high school, Mike Dolan, who was a highly ranked Olympic weight lifter at the time. Under his guidance I made tremendous progress, and had fun doing it. In addition to being a competitive weight lifter I played noseguard and tackle on the high school football team. Being a competitive athlete taught me that hard work yields results, but smart work—that is, putting hard work to the best possible use with efficient, cutting-edge training methods—is better still.

I played college football and studied exercise science at Western State College in Gunnison, Colorado. My adviser there, Karen Jensen, was the person who first informed me about strength and conditioning coach positions, where people got paid to help men and women become fitter and healthier. From that moment onward I was determined to make a career in this field.

Karen also encouraged me to study nutrition, and I gladly began doing so. Meanwhile, as an athlete I had the opportunity to apply everything I was learning. I was able to put together my growing knowledge of nutrition and exercise science with what I loved to do, and establish a solid foundation for my future work.

In the summer after my final year of college, I took up mountain biking and I started to eat better (not only because I now knew how, but also because I didn't have a pass to the cafeteria anymore!). I dropped from my playing weight of 260 pounds all the way down to 225, becoming leaner than I had ever been. I felt great and I liked the changes I saw in my physique. This experience bolstered my appreciation of the importance of leanness in relation to looking and feeling my best.

In 1997 I received a master's degree in exercise and nutrition from Colorado State University. Two years later I became the strength and conditioning coach of the Colorado Avalanche hockey team. Hockey players are tremendous athletes. Working with them has strengthened my belief that "form follows function" when it comes to improving bodies. These guys are very lean, strong, and healthy, and it all comes as a result of the smart methods they use to train for and fuel performance.

Elite athletes come in all shapes and sizes, but the one thing that nearly all of them have in common—from boxers and triathletes to figure skaters and beach volleyball players—is leanness. Sports stars such as golfer Tiger Woods and tennis player Maria Sharapova truly exemplify the "Lean Look." And since top athletes are the leanest people around, doesn't it make sense that nonathletes might borrow their methods to achieve the Lean Look for themselves? It's not as daunting as it sounds. I'm not talking about quitting your job and working out several hours a day. I'm talking about using the most effective nutrition and fitness strategies—those that athletes swear by—and adapting them to your lifestyle.

As the performance director for a new fitness facility in Evergreen, Colorado, I do exactly what I've just described in my work with many nonathletes—men and women of all ages, goals, backgrounds, and starting points. Believe it or not, I use essentially the same approach to help a grandmother improve her mobility or an obese teenager get lean as I use to prepare my hockey players to win another Stanley Cup.

Conditioning and fueling your body for performance is the best way to improve how your body functions not only in sports, but also in life. And it's the best way to improve how you look and feel. Competitive athletes have a lot at stake, so it's vitally important for them to use the most efficient and effective conditioning and nutrition methods out there. They may be willing to spend more time working out than the rest of us, but they are even less willing to waste their time on workouts that aren't giving them maximum results. As a nonathlete you need not copy the conditioning and nutrition methods of competitive athletes in every detail, but you stand to make amazing progress by shifting away from the standard approach of "dieting" and "exercising" and instead focusing on training and fueling for performance, as competitive athletes do.

The Lean Look is an outgrowth of my work in helping everyday men and women achieve the Lean Look using the most effective and efficient methods borrowed from top athletes. The three-phase, 12-week program that I will show you in this book is based on the program that I offer my nonathlete clients. I guarantee it's unlike anything you've tried before. The difference stems from the Lean Look program's explicit goal: to make you lean. Weight loss is only a secondary concern. Before you even begin the program you will learn some fast and easy ways to estimate your body fat percentage, and you will be asked to take an initial measurement of that percentage. You will repeat this process every week throughout the program to track your progress.

A different goal (getting lean instead of "losing weight") requires different methods, and the Lean Look program's methods are unique. The program has three components: a nutrition component, a resistance-training component, and a cardio exercise component. The resistance exercise and cardio exercise components use the athletic principles of variation and progression to coax your fitness level upward (and your body fat level downward) quickly and steadily, and include exercises that can be done either at home or in a gym. The nutrition component, instead of asking you to start over, as most diets do, meets you where you are and requires only that you make a series of small, simple changes that will produce incredible results without the usual deprivations. Trust me: The competitive athletes I work with don't go hungry.

I teamed up with Matt Fitzgerald, a noted fitness author, to write this book because I saw a glaring need for a body transformation program based on measuring and reducing what really matters: body fat percentage. I believe *every* diet and exercise program should have this foundation. Yet the popular diet and exercise programs continue to stubbornly focus on weight and size, ignoring the recent advances that have made self-measurements of body fat percentage as cheap and convenient as using a bathroom scale.

For years my clients have benefited from my program. As I often tell my clients, "A scale doesn't know the difference between one hundred pounds of muscle and one hundred pounds of fat." But it disappoints me that the vast majority of people have not been exposed to this way of thinking and are not even aware that the programs they *have* been exposed to are stuck in the past, chasing the wrong goals with the wrong methods. I wish that I could personally steer every man and woman who is serious about improving his or her body onto the right path of leanness—I am the Dean of Lean, after all—but I trust that this book is the next best thing.

Let's get started!

CHAPTER 1

Why Leaner

Is Better

Do you wish that you were skinny? Would you like to lose weight? Well, guess what? I'm here to help you set a different goal—a better goal. Instead of getting skinny, I want you to get *lean.* Instead of losing weight, I want you to lose *fat,* while gaining muscle. I want you to achieve the Lean Look.

The Lean Look is my name for the tight, toned physique that you get when you lower your body fat percentage by burning away excess body fat stores and strengthening your muscles. It's the outward appearance that you earn through maximizing your inner vitality with a healthy, balanced lifestyle. And it has nothing to do with being skinny.

To be skinny is simply to have a low body weight for your

height. Unlike leanness, skinniness comes primarily from having small muscles and only secondarily from having a small amount of body fat. Since body fat percentage is affected by both muscle mass and fat mass, skinny individuals, who have little of both, are not as lean as those who have small amounts of body fat and strong muscles. In fact, there are some men and women who look skinny but have just as much body fat as people who are obviously overweight. Why is this important? Because science has shown that skinny individuals are not as healthy as lean ones. Doctors recently coined the term normal weight obese to categorize men and women who fall within the normal body weight range but have more than 30 percent body fat. Studies have found that normal weight obese individuals have the same levels of circulating inflammation markers—a major risk factor for heart disease—as do those who are technically obese.

In recent years medical researchers have performed a number of studies comparing the effect of body weight versus body composition (or body fat percentage) on the risk for various diseases. The conclusion is always the same. While heavier men and women do have a higher risk for lifestyle diseases such as heart disease than do normal-weight men and women, the connection between body fat percentage and disease risk is much stronger. In fact, heavier individuals with a low body fat percentage tend to be healthier and to live longer than skinnier individuals with a higher body fat percentage.

Why is having even a little excess body fat so damaging to our health? It appears that excess body fat contributes to a slew of different diseases via various mechanisms. For example, high levels of abdominal fat are associated with high levels of low-density lipoprotein (LDL) cholesterol in the blood— and the more LDL cholesterol there is in the blood, the faster it accumulates in the arterial plaques, establishing the basis of heart disease.

A second reason that lean men and women are healthier than their skinny counterparts has to do with muscle. Recent medical research has shown that muscle mass is as beneficial to health as excess body fat is damaging to health. Having a little extra muscle has been shown to increase metabolism, reduce insulin resistance and diabetes risk, increase bone density and lower the risk of osteoporosis, and more. Having a little extra muscle even increases longevity. A number of studies have found that, among elderly populations, those with the most muscle strength live the longest.

What's more, research in the field of psychology has demonstrated that lean bodies (such as those of top athletes) are almost universally considered to be more attractive than skinny bodies (such as those of many fashion models) in both women and men. The muscle tone that comes with the Lean Look gives both male and female bodies a contoured appearance that is quite distinct from the straight-up-and-down look of skinniness. Several psychologists, including Devendra Singh at the University of Texas, have found that men consistently show a preference for a curvy, athletic form rather than the narrow, linear shape of skinny women, while women clearly prefer a moderate, fit-looking male physique to lanky ones, fat ones, and even extremely muscular ones.

JUST SAY "NO" TO DIETING

I realize that skinniness is not the major health problem in our society. Fatness is. But the reason I've taken such pains to distinguish leanness from skinniness is that when people set a goal to simply lose weight or get skinny, they usually pursue this goal by dieting. The trouble with dieting is that it is difficult to sustain, and even when a diet does last, it fails to improve one's health or appearance as much as a program that is tailored to achieving leanness.

Surveys show that a majority of men and women who try to lose weight do so by cutting way back on the number of calories they eat (and usually not exercising). In most cases they choose to follow a popular branded diet such as South Beach, Weight Watchers, or the Atkins Diet. On the surface these diets seem very different. One tells you to virtually eliminate carbs from your diet, another tells you to keep the carbs and eliminate fat instead, and still another encourages you to get most of your calories from processed drink mixes and food bars. But beneath the surface almost all of these eating plans are essentially the same thing: low-calorie diets.

Now, I won't deny the fact that in order to shed body fat most people have to reduce the number of calories they consume each day. However, there is a big difference between merely trimming calories, as I will have you do in the Lean Look program, and going on a low-calorie diet, as most popular diets require. The difference is that merely trimming calories is easy and painless, whereas low-calorie diets are unpleasant and therefore very difficult to sustain. Low-calorie diets demand high levels of restraint when it comes to eat-

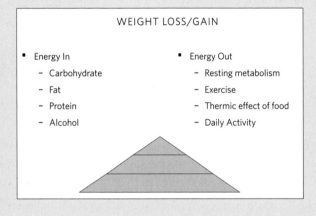

THE ENERGY BALANCING ACT

Whether you lose or gain weight depends on whether your body uses more energy than it consumes or consumes more energy than it uses. This illustration shows the factors that affect both sides of the energy balance.

WEIGHT LOSS/GAIN

- Energy In
  - Carbohydrate
  - Fat
  - Protein
  - Alcohol

- Energy Out
  - Resting metabolism
  - Exercise
  - Thermic effect of food
  - Daily Activity

ing and force the dieter to live with persistent hunger. When you go on a low-calorie diet, suddenly many of your favorite foods are off-limits. Your meals are too small to satisfy your hunger for very long, if at all. As a result, you end up being distracted by your rumbling stomach and thinking about food—especially your favorite off-limits foods—most of the day. It's only a matter of time before you scream, "To hell with it!" and break the diet. Surveys have shown that the average weight-loss diet lasts just two weeks!

Because dieters are rarely able to sustain their low-calorie eating plans (and frequently wind up eating even more than normal after they break the diet), the rapid weight loss they experience in the first days and weeks of the diet is followed by rapid weight gain of equal or greater amount. More often than not, this failure motivates the dieter to try again. Consequently, many dieters engage in a repeating cycle of rapid weight loss followed by rapid weight gain (called *weight cycling,* or *yo-yo dieting)* that is especially harmful. For reasons that are not yet fully understood, weight cycling increases the risk of cardiovascular disease and all-cause mortality (death by any cause) beyond the level associated with any given degree of overweight. One possible explanation is that yo-yo dieters actually worsen their body composition by regaining less muscle and more fat than they initially lost while dieting.

Even when it does not lead to weight cycling, dieting almost always results in substantial loss of muscle and water, along with fat, and therefore does little to improve body composition. Severe calorie restriction is basically a form of semistarvation, and under starvation conditions the body breaks down almost as much muscle protein for energy as it does body fat. The problem of muscle loss during dieting is compounded by the fact that severe calorie restriction provides little energy for exercise, which is indispensable to improving body composition. Indeed, few dieters even bother with exercise. One survey found that less than a third of men and women who said they were "trying" to lose weight engaged in regular exercise. Talk about setting yourself up for failure!

The path to leanness is a lot healthier, more enjoyable, and more sustainable than dieting to become skinny. The best way to get lean is to starve not your whole body, as in dieting, but only your body fat stores, while at the same time fully nourishing your muscles. You can do this quite easily by (1) eating more foods that promote muscle development, (2) cutting back on foods that promote fat storage, (3) timing your meals to promote muscle development and prevent fat storage, (4) exercising to burn body fat, and (5) exercising to develop muscle tone. Only a combination of healthy eating and exercise—which is the essence of the Lean Look program—can truly optimize your body composition.

WHAT GETS MEASURED GETS MANAGED

I just listed five factors—five elements of the Lean Look program—that promote leanness. There is actually a sixth factor, a sort of wild card, which helps to promote leanness in a different way. I'm talking about monitoring your leanness by taking regular body fat measurements.

In the corporate world many senior executives are fond of the expression "What gets measured gets managed." I like this expression, too, and I think it applies to health and fitness. If you want to gain greater control over some aspect of your business (or your body), one of the best things you can do is to monitor it systematically using some kind of measuring stick. The very effort you take to do so makes it a higher priority and helps you improve this aspect of your business or your body independently of other efforts (such as the five ways of promoting leanness I have already listed).

In the Lean Look program you will be encouraged to measure your body fat percentage regularly using either of two simple and affordable methods described in the next chapter: a body fat scale or the tape measure method. You can also try an even simpler alternative to these methods—measuring the circumference of your waist, which provides a less exact but still helpful indication of leanness. Measuring your body fat percentage will help you manage it better by providing proof of your progress and thereby increasing your motivation and the amount of effort you put into the program.

If you're not the measuring type and prefer to just launch into the Lean Look program and observe the results in the mirror—something you will have no difficulty doing (the results you see in the mirror may be your most gratifying result even if you do use a body fat scale)—that's okay. But if you're open to fully committing to the management of your body by measuring your leanness on a regular basis, I believe you will be well rewarded for the small effort it takes.

WHAT IS A "GOOD" BODY FAT PERCENTAGE?

So, if being lean is good, and if body fat percentage is a good indicator of leanness, what is a good body fat percentage? There is no specific body fat percentage that is optimal for everyone. Age, gender, genetics, and other factors all play a part in determining the body fat percentage that is ideal for you at any given time. The most important variables are age and gender. The average woman needs and has more body fat than the average man. Also, body fat percentage naturally increases with age. If you're over fifty you should not expect to be able to get quite as lean as a twenty-two-year-old can.

Scientists have come up with age- and gender-based healthy body fat percentage ranges based on correlations between various body fat percentages and risk for diseases linked to excess body fat. The following chart presents a set of proposed healthy body fat percentage ranges that were published in the *American Journal of Clinical Nutrition*. I have a personal objection to the low end of these ranges, because I routinely deal with female athletes with less than 20 percent body fat and male athletes with less than 8 percent body fat who are about as healthy as a human being can be. But one thing is certain: If your current body fat percentage is outside the healthy range for your age and gender *on the high end,* you need to lower it!

HEALTHY BODY FAT PERCENTAGE RANGES

AGE	HEALTHY BODY FAT PERCENTAGE FOR WOMEN	HEALTHY BODY FAT PERCENTAGE FOR MEN
20-39	21-32	8-19
40-59	23-33	11-21
60-79	24-35	13-24

Source: American Journal of Clinical Nutrition

The body fat percentage you are able to achieve after completing the Lean Look program may or may not be your personal optimum level for your present age. If you are already fairly lean, there's a good chance that you will achieve your optimal body fat percentage by the end of the program. If you are not already fairly lean, then it could take a lot longer. But don't worry—in chapter 16 I show you how to extend the Lean Look program so that you can continue to make progress until you reach your personal body composition goal.

It is not possible to predict exactly what your personal optimal body fat percentage will turn out to be. You just have to continue eating right, exercising, and measuring your body fat and see where you end up. Your body fat measurements will continue to go down as you approach your ideal body composition and will eventually level off when you get there. At that time, as long as you're still adhering to the Lean Look lifestyle, you can trust that you have truly achieved your best body.

CHAPTER 2

How to Measure Your Leanness

The device I use to analyze body composition with my hands-on clients is called the Bod Pod. It looks a lot like Mork's egg from the old *Mork and Mindy* television show. I like it not only because it is quite accurate but also because, unlike most other methods of measuring body composition, the Bod Pod provides consistent results regardless of the tester. There's no possibility for error or individual variation among different testers because all you have to do to operate the device is press a button. But before you rush out and buy a Bod Pod, you should know that the basic model costs $20,000 and the top-end model goes for $70,000!

Fortunately there are two fairly accurate ways you can use to measure your body fat percentage affordably and conveniently on the Lean Look program: with a body fat scale or using the tape measure method.

BODY FAT SCALES

Body fat scales using bioelectrical impedance technology are now widely available at department stores, drugstores, sporting goods stores, and elsewhere. In fact, the recent explosion in sales of these devices is one of the major reasons I decided to write this book. I have relied on body fat testing with my own clients for many years, but until recently I didn't think that accurate self-testing was convenient or affordable enough that I could offer my program to a mass audience. Now these devices are accurate enough to depend on for this program and are as easy to use, easy to find and affordable as a bathroom scale.

When used properly, body fat scales produce more accurate results than the tape measure method discussed in the next section; the latter is the only cheaper way to get body fat measurements. Indeed, a study published in the *Clinical Journal of Nutrition* found that devices using bioelectrical impedance were nearly as accurate as isotope dilution (a clinical method involving the injection of "tracers" into the bloodstream) and more accurate than skinfold measurements. Body fat scales with this degree of accuracy are available for as little as $40.

Body fat scales look just like regular bathroom scales. You step onto one and get a measurement. And they do in fact measure your body weight in addition to estimating your body fat percentage. Body fat scales work by sending an electrical signal into your body and measuring the degree of resistance (or impedance) the signal encounters in your body. Electrical signals pass through fat tissue more quickly than they do through muscle tissue, so the less resistance the body fat scale registers, the higher your body fat percentage must be.

To ensure accurate results, it is important that you use your device in strict accordance with the instructions included with it. Different units have slightly different requirements. Here are some usage guidelines that apply to all body fat scales:

1. Always measure your body fat at the same time of day, preferably at least two hours after eating.
2. Make sure that you are well hydrated.
3. Use the bathroom before stepping on the scale.
4. Moisten a towel and step on it with bare feet before stepping on the scale (to enhance conductivity).
5. Make sure the scale is on a flat, hard surface (such as bathroom tiles).
6. If you have good reason to believe that your body fat percentage is already low (e.g., you have visible abdominal musculature), purchase a scale with an "athlete" mode, such as the Tanita Ironman series. Scales without this feature are less accurate for lean individuals.

Body fat scales range in price from $40 to $150. The difference between the higher-priced body fat scales and the cheaper models is mainly in the number of features, not their accuracy. For example, some of the pricier athlete-oriented units measure hydration level in addition to body weight and body fat percentage. You can find body fat scales at department stores, drugstores, and sporting goods stores. (See Appendix C for a list of popular brands.)

THE TAPE MEASURE METHOD

The U.S. military has recognized for many years that body fat percentage is a much more useful indicator of health and fitness than is body weight. For this reason there is no maximum permissible body weight for acceptance into the armed forces, but there is a maximum body fat percentage. The Army, Marines, and Navy require that all personnel remain below this limit for the duration of their careers.

Because universal body composition testing was instituted before the development of newer methods that are now cheap, fast, *and* accurate, the military developed its own tape measure method to estimate body fat percentage. For men, the circumference of the waist and neck are measured and these measurements, plus height, are run through a complex calculation. For women there is one additional circumference measurement at the hips.

The tape measure method is accurate for most people. But it is not accurate for individuals who are very lean (men below 9 percent body fat and women below 19 percent body fat), nor is it accurate for individuals who are skinny and not particularly lean (i.e., the normal weight obese). If you fall into either of these categories, you should probably use a body fat scale instead. Also, as you become leaner through the Lean Look program and beyond, the tape measure method may become less and less accurate for you, because the pools of subjects used to create the calculations this method employs did not include a lot of super-lean individuals.

You can take the circumference measurements yourself or have a partner take them. Perform all of the measurements without clothing, if possible. Women using a partner to do the measurements may, of course, have the hip circumference measurement taken while wearing light clothing. Take each measurement three times and average the results. Use a pen to mark each spot on your body where the first measurement is taken so you can easily find exactly the same spot again for the second and third measurements. Here's how to do the measurements:

MEN

Neck: Have a partner take this measurement, or do it standing in front of a mirror. Using a fabric tape measure (available wherever sewing supplies are sold), measure the circumference of your neck just below the Adam's apple. Round the measurement up to the nearest half inch.

Waist: Measure the circumference of your waist at the level of your navel after exhaling. Do not suck in your stomach. (I mean it!) Round the measurement up to the nearest half inch.

WOMEN

Neck: Have a partner take this measurement, or do it standing in front of a mirror. Using a fabric tape measure, measure the circumference of your neck just below the voice box. Round the measurement up to the nearest half inch.

Waist. Measure the circumference of your waist at the narrowest point, which in most women is halfway between the navel and the bottom of the rib cage. Exhale before taking the measurement and do not suck in your stomach. Round the measurement down to the nearest half inch.

Hips. Measure the circumference of your hips at their broadest point (the level of the buttocks' greatest protrusion). If a partner takes this measurement and you wear clothing for it, wear the lightest clothing possible and have the measurer apply enough tension to the tape measure to minimize the effects of the clothing. Round down to the nearest half inch.

In addition to these circumference measurements, you also need to know your height in inches to calculate your body fat percentage using this method. Since the math required is somewhat complex, I have made tables of all possible results, which you'll find in Appendix A. Here's how to use them:

Men. Subtract your neck measurement from your waist measurement and look up the result on the correct chart for your height.

Women. Add your waist and hip measurements together, subtract your neck measurement from the sum, and then look up this number on the correct chart for your height.

Consistency is vital to ensuring the accuracy of the results you get from the tape measure method. If you have a partner take your circumference measurements the first time, have the same partner take them every time thereafter. If you begin with self-measurement, stay with self-measurement.

12 WEEKS, 13 MEASUREMENTS

You will take 13 body fat measurements in the 12-week Lean Look program. Start with a "before" measurement taken one day, or at most a few days, before you start the program. Then take progress measurements at the end of each week, including a final measurement at the end of week 12. If you adhere to the program faithfully throughout the 12 weeks, you will see a significant drop in your body fat percentage. Resist the temptation to take measurements more often than once a week—your body fat percentage won't go down much from one day to the next no matter how well you're doing.

While your chosen method of body fat measurement will give you objective proof of your body transformation, there will be plenty of other evidence. You will look leaner and healthier to yourself and everyone else, you will be physically fitter, and you will *feel* better: more energetic, more confident, and less stressed. These are the results that really count. Body fat measurements are just a tool to help you achieve them.

ANOTHER OPTION

If you would rather not spend $50 or so for a body fat scale and the tape measure method looks a little too complicated, there is another option: waist circumference measurements. Waist circumference measurements provide a fairly true indication of leanness, although they are not nearly precise enough to provide a useful body fat percentage estimate. The purpose of taking waist circumference measurements throughout the Lean Look program would simply be to provide quantitative evidence of progress without going to the expense of buying a body fat scale or the effort of using the tape measure method.

All you have to do is wrap a cloth tape measure snugly around your waist just above the crest of your hipbones and take a reading. Do this before you start the Lean Look program and again once a week throughout the program as an alternative to measuring your body fat percentage.

Naturally, as you lose inches off your waist you will be able to see improvements in the look of your body when looking in the mirror. If this type of evidence is all you really care about, you should not feel obligated to take any other measurements of any sort on the Lean Look program. The truly indispensable components of the program are the nutrition guidelines and the resistance and cardio workouts. These were designed to produce the greatest possible improvement in leanness without undue sacrifice. By following the 12-week program you will transform your body dramatically for the better whether you take measurements or not.

CHAPTER 3

An Overview of the Lean Look Program

The number one reason diets end in failure is the inability to keep up the required restrictions. The number one reason people don't exercise is lack of time. The Lean Look program offers a solution to these common roadblocks to achieving your best body. It stipulates very few dietary restrictions and involves an efficient, easily accommodated fitness component.

The basic Lean Look plan is twelve weeks long and consists of three phases of four weeks each. But after the twelve weeks are over you can expand the program and repeat it in a progressive manner for ongoing progress. I share how to do this in chapter 16 ("Lean for Life").

The program features three components: nutrition, resistance exercise, and cardio (or fat-burning) exercise. Each component evolves from one phase to the next. Your resistance-training regimen in Phase II builds on your resistance-training regimen in Phase I, and your resistance-training regimen in Phase III builds on your resistance-training regimen in Phase II. The same pattern holds for the cardio and nutrition components.

THE NUTRITION COMPONENT

Achieving optimal leanness, fitness, and health requires both healthy eating and consistent exercise. But if I had to pick which of these two essential components comes first, I would have to pick healthy eating. Nutrition is like the soil a plant grows in. Exercise is like the sun and watering that help it grow. While adequate sunlight and watering are needed for healthy growth, a plant won't even sprout from its seed if it's planted in the wrong soil.

Similarly, healthy eating is the true foundation for leanness, fitness, and health. Exercise won't get you anywhere if you don't nourish your body properly. For this reason I discuss the nutrition component of the Lean Look program before the resistance and cardio exercise components.

In the nutrition component of Phase I you will make a number of small, calorie-cutting substitutions in your food choices and nutrition habits. Each of these substitutions will assist in feeding and fueling your muscles while producing the opposite effect on your body fat stores. Notice I say "substitutions" instead of "restrictions." Replacing poor food choices with better ones is a much better strategy for improving your diet than simply saying "no" to poor food choices. In all there are only ten key substitutions you may need to make (depending on your current eating habits).

Phase II is all about nutrient timing—a powerful way to enhance leanness without cutting calories, based on exciting new scientific research. In chapter 9, which is devoted to the topic of nutrient timing, I will show you how to make better use of the calories you eat by taking in the right types of nutrients at the right time of day, using the eight tips I provide here. My clients are amazed by the impact that simply changing *when* they eat has on their performance and body composition.

In Phase III we will discuss several supplements you can use to take your performance and leanness to the next level. I'm not the biggest supplements advocate. But there is a small handful of supplements that have been proven effective by sound science and work very well with my clients, and I think you should know about them. I will also tell you which supplements to avoid.

The three phases of the Lean Look program's nutrition component are additive. The ten key substitutions are introduced in Phase I and maintained in Phases II and III. The eight nutrient timing practices are added in Phase II and are continued in Phase III. Finally, any smart supplements you may care to try are added in Phase III.

Why is the nutrition component of the Lean Look program separated into three phases? Couldn't you start practicing calorie-cutting food substitutions, nutrient timing, and smart supplementation simultaneously at the beginning of Phase I? You could. However, unless you are powerfully motivated to do so, I recommend that you follow the suggested phase progression. The rationale for separating the nutrition component of the Lean Look program into separate phases is that people attempting to make positive lifestyle changes often become overwhelmed and burn out quickly when they attempt to make too many drastic changes too quickly. I want you to avoid this pitfall, so the Lean Look program will have you make only the most important diet changes—key substitutions—in the first four weeks, and then incorporate changes in your nutrient timing in the next four weeks, and finally introduce smart supplementation in the final four weeks of the program.

THE RESISTANCE EXERCISE COMPONENT

Resistance exercise is an important complement to cardio exercise. The essence of resistance exercise is contracting your muscles against strong resistance. Whether the source of resistance is your own body weight, dumbbells, an elastic cable, or something else, the benefits are the same. Resistance exercise promotes the Lean Look in three ways.

1. Resistance workouts burn a lot of calories (not only during but even after the workouts). While they don't burn quite as many calories as do cardio workouts, they still burn plenty, especially if you do circuit workouts, as you will in the Lean Look program. (I'll say more about the circuit format for resistance workouts momentarily.) And the more calories you burn in a day

through activity, the more fat you will lose, assuming you are also eating as you should.

2. Resistance workouts also cause *hypertrophy,* or growth of the muscles. Even a small amount of muscle growth can have a dramatic effect on the shape of your individual body parts and your overall physique. Well-toned muscles have a firm look and attractive contours. Resistance exercise therefore enhances the *appearance* of leanness above and beyond its effects on your body fat percentage.

3. Resistance exercise also promotes fat loss in an indirect way. The amount of food calories that are required to maintain a pound of muscle each day is between 15 and 25 times greater than the number required to maintain a pound of fat. In other words, muscle tissue is a total energy hog compared to adipose (fat) tissue. So as you gain muscle mass, you increase the number of calories your body burns each day, even when you are at rest. Put another way, getting leaner itself actually helps you get even leaner.

Resistance exercise is associated with a wide range of health benefits. It reduces insulin resistance, abdominal fat storage, and blood pressure—three risk factors for diabetes, heart disease, stroke, and heart attack. Resistance exercise enhances strength, mobility, stability, and performance in activities of daily living, such as opening pickle jars and lifting heavy boxes. It increases bone density, lowering the risk of osteoporosis and fractures, and certain exercises also prevent and treat lower back pain—a condition that affects more than 60 percent of adults at some point in their lives. Look forward to achieving all of these benefits through the Lean Look program's resistance-training component.

The secret to getting the greatest muscle conditioning results from the least amount of resistance exercise is the circuit workout format. In a circuit workout you continually move from one exercise to the next with minimal rest in between. By minimizing rest between exercises you keep your heart rate and caloric burn rate high, producing greater fat loss and greater cardiovascular benefit to go along with the muscle conditioning effect of the workout. Circuit training originated with elite athletes and remains a staple in the training programs I prescribe for competitive athletes.

One of the original studies on the effects of circuit training found that it produced substantial improvements in both strength and body composition.

And in a more recent Finnish study, sedentary adults who completed a twelve-week circuit-training program improved their cardiovascular fitness as much as controls who walked, jogged, cycled, and skied cross-country, while also improving their strength. The circuit-training workout is the ultimate "two-for-one" workout.

In the Lean Look program you'll do a wide variety of resistance exercises and three distinct types of resistance workouts to provide the consistent challenge that is needed to experience consistent gains. You'll also progress from easily managed circuits to more and more challenging workouts as your fat mass plummets.

The art and science of breaking up your fitness program into distinct phases, each emphasizing a different type of training, is called *periodization*. Competitive athletes use periodization routinely to achieve better results, and it will do the same for you in the Lean Look program. In Phase I your resistance workouts will feature muscle-balancing exercises. These are simple exercises designed to strengthen muscles evenly throughout the body, with special attention given to problem areas that tend to be especially underdeveloped in most Americans (for example, the lower back and the lower abdominal area). It is very important to develop muscle balance before you move on to more advanced types of resistance exercise. Conditioning the muscles is like building a house—you have to start with a solid foundation. Muscle balancing is the foundation of the overall muscle-conditioning process.

Phase II emphasizes multi-joint exercises (i.e., exercises involving movement at more than one joint and activation of multiple muscle groups) that build strength in functional movements. These more advanced exercises build on the muscle balance you have achieved in the previous phase and produce visible improvements in muscle tone very quickly.

In Phase III, power exercises—exercises that build a combination of strength and speed—are added to the mix. Power exercises challenge your muscles in a slightly different way than do conventional strength exercises. Adding power exercises to the program keeps the "adaptive momentum" going so your muscles continue to develop even after they have become somewhat accustomed to conventional strength exercises. *Adaptive momentum* is a state where your muscles are always ready to respond to a new challenge, because the one thing you've allowed them to get used to is new workout challenges.

Each phase of the resistance exercise component of the Lean Look program presents a large pool of exercises that can be drawn from to create complete circuit workouts. The equipment needed to perform these exercises is minimal, so you can work out at home if you prefer. I will outline the specific equipment options in chapter 6. Each resistance workout takes no more than 30 minutes to complete on the beginner schedule, and no more than 39 minutes on the advanced schedule.

As I've just mentioned, you have the choice of two separate resistance workout levels to follow on the Lean Look program: beginner and advanced. Both levels feature the same frequency and types of workouts, but those on the advanced level include more total exercises per workout. Throughout the program you will do three resistance workouts per week, on Monday, Wednesday, and Friday.

THE CARDIO EXERCISE COMPONENT

The most effective forms of exercise for fat burning and enhancing general health are those that involve sustained movement, such as jogging, bicycling, and swimming. Collectively these forms of exercise are known as aerobic or cardiovascular exercise—or cardio exercise. During cardio exercise many of your body's normal functions speed up dramatically: your heart pumps more blood, your lungs absorb more oxygen, and your muscles break down more fuel stores (mainly fat and carbohydrates) for energy. As you know, the energy that comes from nutrients is measured in calories. Thus by greatly increasing the demand for nutrient energy, cardio exercise causes your body to burn calories at many times the rate it burns them when you are at rest.

Speeding up your natural body processes through cardio exercise on a consistent basis results in a long list of healthy adaptations. The most obvious one is fat loss. In fact, research has shown that cardio exercise is the single most powerful predictor of success in maintaining a healthy body weight. In other words, men and women who participate in regular cardio exercise are more likely to stay lean than those who follow any kind of diet (low-fat, low-carb, vegetarian, or whatever) but do not work out consistently. Yet cardio exercise does much more than help you burn off excess body fat. It is also proven to help prevent heart disease, heart attack, stroke, diabetes, high blood pressure, Alzheimer's disease, and cancer. It strengthens the immune system, reduces stress, enhances self-esteem, reduces depressive symptoms, strengthens antioxidant defenses and thereby slows the aging process, increases life span, and even improves memory and other mental functions. In summary, there's very little that cardio exercise *doesn't* do.

The secret to getting the greatest fat-burning results from the least amount of cardio exercise is interval workouts and variation. Interval workouts consist of short (or relatively short) segments of high-intensity activity separated by low-intensity "active recovery" periods. These workouts burn fat and boost cardiovascular fitness faster than do slow and steady cardio workouts. Slow and steady cardio workouts are effective too, but they are not nearly as time-efficient as well-designed interval workouts. Interval workouts are also proven to increase the body's metabolism (i.e., calorie burning) after exercise compared to slow and steady cardio workouts.

The second key to cardio training, in addition to intervals, is variation. The principle of variation states that results come faster when you challenge your body through exercise in various ways instead of doing basically the same workout every time. Perhaps the most obvious difference between the way most people exercise and the way top athletes train is that athletes include much more variation in their programs. And this key difference is one of the main reasons for the better results they get. I rely heavily on the principle of variation in my hands-on work with clients. One thing they all learn is that they will never know exactly what I will have them do the next time they see me (even though I have it all planned out). The Lean Look program is highly varied. And because of this, you will get better, faster results from less workout time.

Put intervals and variation together and you get varied interval workouts. Separate the various types of interval workouts into distinct phases and you get a periodized approach to cardio training that is more effective than any alternative. That's the essence of the Lean Look program's cardio component. Phase I emphasizes three types of short intervals (20-second, 30-second, and 1-minute), which are the best way for those just beginning an exercise program to get fast results without overexerting themselves. Phase II emphasizes intermediate intervals (2- and 3-minute intervals), which help you to build on the fitness gains made in Phase I with short intervals. Phase III adds long intervals (4- and 6-minute intervals) to the mix. My clients use these sustained intervals to take their cardio fitness and leanness to peak levels, and so will you.

The Lean Look program does not require that you use any particular form of cardio exercise. Choose your favorite. These intervals work with all of them. In chapter 7 I will discuss the advantages and disadvantages of six types of cardio training—bicycling, elliptical training and stair climbing, inline skating, running, swimming, and walking—and how to get started in each.

Like the resistance exercise component, the cardio exercise component offers two separate workout schedules: beginner and advanced. Both schedules feature the same frequency and types of workouts, but the advanced schedule contains more intervals and therefore takes slightly longer to complete. Throughout the program you will do three cardio workouts per week, on Tuesday, Thursday, and Saturday. Sunday is a rest day.

THE 12-WEEK LEAN LOOK RESISTANCE AND CARDIO WORKOUT SCHEDULE

The following chart presents a general Lean Look exercise schedule that includes resistance and cardio workouts and combines the beginner and advanced schedules. If you look at the estimated workout duration range at the bottom of each box, the number at the low end of the range represents the duration of that workout on the beginner schedule and the number at the high end of the range represents the duration of the advanced version of that same workout. You will find separate and more detailed workout schedules for the three phases in the introduction to each phase and specific workout guidelines in the individual chapters dealing with the resistance exercise component and cardio exercise component of each phase.

Should you follow the beginner or the advanced workout schedule? If you have not been working out regularly in recent weeks or months, or if you have little strength-training experience, or you just feel more comfortable starting with gentler workouts, use the beginner schedule. If you have at least a modest baseline of fitness or prefer to enjoy the faster results that will come from a more challenging workout regimen, choose the advanced schedule. You can switch from one schedule to the other if necessary at any time after you've started the program.

Wk #	Monday	Tuesday	Wednesday	Thursday	Friday	Saturday
1	Resistance (Muscle Balancing) 12–15 minutes	Cardio (Speed Intervals) 15–18 minutes	Resistance (Muscle Balancing) 12–15 minutes	Cardio (1-Minute Intervals) 17–21 minutes	Resistance (Muscle Balancing) 12–15 minutes	Cardio (Power Intervals) 18–23 minutes
2	Resistance (Muscle Balance) 12–15 minutes	Cardio (Speed Intervals) 17–20 minutes	Resistance (Muscle Balance) 12–15 minutes	Cardio (1-Minute Intervals) 19–23 minutes	Resistance (Muscle Balance) 12–15 minutes	Cardio (Power Intervals) 21–26 minutes
3	Resistance (Muscle Balancing) 21–27 minutes	Cardio (Speed Intervals) 18–21 minutes	Resistance (Muscle Balancing) 21–27 minutes	Cardio (1-Minute Intervals) 21–25 minutes	Resistance (Muscle Balancing) 21–27minutes	Cardio (Power Intervals) 23–28 minutes
4	Resistance (Muscle Balancing) 12–15 minutes	Cardio (Speed Intervals) 15–18 minutes	Resistance (Muscle Balancing) 12–15 minutes	Cardio (1-Minute Intervals) 17–21 minutes	Resistance (Muscle Balancing) 12–15 minutes	Cardio (Power Intervals) 18–23 minutes
5	Resistance (Strength) 21–27 minutes	Cardio (2-Minute Intervals) 24–28 minutes	Resistance (Muscle Balancing) 21–27 minutes	(1-Minute Intervals) 21–25 minutes	Resistance (Strength) 21–27 minutes	Cardio (3-Minute Intervals) 25–31 minutes
6	Resistance (Strength) 30–39 minutes	Cardio (2-Minute Intervals) 28–32 minutes	Resistance (Muscle Balancing) 30–39 minutes	Cardio (1-Minute Intervals) 23–27 minutes	Resistance (Strength) 30–39 minutes	Cardio (3-Minute Intervals) 25–31 minutes

    The phrases that appear between parentheses in the above chart refer to the specific type of resistance or cardio interval workout scheduled for that day. For example, "Muscle Balancing" denotes a muscle-balancing resistance workout, while "1-Minute Intervals" denotes a cardio workout featuring repeated 1-minute intervals. These terms won't mean much to you now, but the workouts they refer to will be fully explained within each phase section.

Wk #	Monday	Tuesday	Wednesday	Thursday	Friday	Saturday
7	Resistance (Strength) 30–39 minutes	Cardio (2-Minute Intervals) 28–32 minutes	Resistance (Muscle Balancing) 30–39 minutes	Cardio (1-Minute Intervals) 25–29 minutes	Resistance (Strength) 30–39 minutes	Cardio (3-Minute Intervals) 31–37 minutes
8	Resistance (Strength) 21–27 minutes	Cardio (2-Minute Intervals) 24–28 minutes	Resistance (Muscle Balancing) 21–27 minutes	Cardio (1-Minute Intervals) 21–25 minutes	Resistance (Strength) 21–27 minutes	Cardio (3-Minute Intervals) 25–31 minutes
9	Resistance (Strength) 18–24 minutes	Cardio (6-Minute Intervals) 25–34 minutes	Resistance (Power) 18–24 minutes	Cardio (2-Minute Intervals) 20–24 minutes	Resistance (Strength) 18–24 minutes	Cardio (4-Minute Intervals) 20–26 minutes
10	Resistance (Strength) 30–39 minutes	Cardio (6-Minute Intervals) 25–34 minutes	Resistance (Power) 30–39 minutes	Cardio (3-Minute Intervals) 25–31 minutes	Resistance (Strength) 30–39 minutes	Cardio (4-Minute Intervals) 26–32 minutes
11	Resistance (Strength) 30–39 minutes	Cardio (6-Minute Intervals) 34–43 minutes	Resistance (Power) 30–39 minutes	Cardio (2-Minute Intervals) 24–28 minutes	Resistance (Strength) 30–39 minutes	Cardio (4-Minute Intervals) 26–32 minutes
12	Resistance (Strength) 21–27 minutes	Cardio (6-Minute Intervals) 25–34 minutes	Resistance (Power) 21–27 minutes	Cardio (3-Minute Intervals) 25–31 minutes	Resistance (Strength) 21–27 minutes	Cardio (4-Minute Intervals) 20–26 minutes

ARE YOU READY?

I have said that the Lean Look program has three phases, but there is also an unofficial fourth phase, which we can call Phase 0. One of the keys to success in any nutrition and exercise program is not starting it before you're ready. In order to be truly ready you have to be emotionally psyched up for success, you need a goal and a plan, you need to understand the rationale behind everything you're doing in the program, and you need to have figured out some practical issues such as when and where you will work out. In other words, you need to look before you leap.

Phase 0 of the Lean Look program consists of reading the rest of this book. Doing so will help you get ready to start the program in all of the ways just mentioned. As eager as you may be to just get started, I encourage you to finish reading first. Although you may need to wait a few days before you embark on Phase I, the delay will be worth it because by waiting and absorbing the text you will be greatly increasing your chances of experiencing long-term success.

PHASE I

CHAPTER 4

Introduction

to Phase I

In Phase I of the Lean Look program you will begin doing six short workouts per week—three resistance workouts and three cardio workouts—and making key food substitutions to trim calories from your diet. Although this phase is only four weeks long, in the course of that time you will achieve a measurable improvement in your body fat percentage—without feeling deprived in your diet or overwhelmed by long workouts.

NUTRITION: KEY FOOD SUBSTITUTIONS

You can achieve substantial fat loss by trimming a relatively small number of calories—between 100 and 300—from your daily diet.

What's more, you can do so without even bothering to count the number of calories you're eating or cutting. All you have to do is modify the meals and snacks you're already eating by making ten key food substitutions, which I'll outline in chapter 5.

RESISTANCE EXERCISE: MUSCLE BALANCING

When you start a new resistance exercise program, your first priority is to gradually habituate your tendons and other connective tissues to the stress of bearing and pulling against great resistance. You must also teach your brain and muscles to "talk" to each other more efficiently—that is, to enhance what is known as *neuromuscular coordination*. And, finally, you have to begin the process of increasing the strength of your many muscles, especially those muscles that are weakest.

The resistance workouts in Phase I of the Lean Look program are made up of exercises that are designed to achieve these important early objectives. I refer to these workouts as "muscle-balancing" resistance workouts. In Weeks 1 and 2 you will perform just one circuit of either 9 (beginner) or 12 (advanced) exercises in each session. In Week 3 you will advance to two circuits, and in the final week of Phase I you will go back down to one circuit to allow your body the opportunity to fully absorb and adapt to the work you've done.

CARDIO EXERCISE: SHORT INTERVALS

Unlike the resistance exercise component of Phase I, which features one specific workout type—muscle-balancing exercises—the cardio component features three distinct types of interval workouts: the speed interval, the power interval, and the 1-minute interval. The speed interval workout features 30-second intervals of very high intensity. The power interval workout features 20-second maximum-intensity intervals performed against high resistance. And the 1-minute interval workout features 1-minute intervals at a slightly lower but still high intensity. You'll do one workout of each type per week throughout Phase I.

The number of intervals you do within each workout will increase from week to week until Week 4, when your cardio workouts will shrink back to their Week 1 level to allow your body to fully absorb and adapt to the work you've done. The speed, power, and 1-minute interval workouts on the advanced schedule contain more intervals than do those on the beginner schedule, so choose what feels right for you. You'll learn more about these cardio workouts in chapter 6.

WORKOUT SCHEDULES

The following charts list the beginner and advanced resistance and cardio workout schedules for Phase I of the Lean Look program. Every step and detail of the Phase I exercises and workouts will be explained in chapters 6 and 7. After you have read through all of Phase I, refer back to the tables provided here, which show you how the resistance and cardio workouts fit together week by week.

BEGINNER SCHEDULE

Wk #	Monday	Tuesday	Wednesday	Thursday	Friday	Saturday
1	Resistance (Muscle Balancing) 1 circuit 9 exercises 9 minutes	Cardio (Speed Intervals) 4 intervals 15 minutes	Resistance (Muscle Balancing) 1 circuit 9 exercises 9 minutes	Cardio (1-Minute Intervals) 4 intervals 17 minutes	Resistance (Muscle Balancing) 1 circuit 9 exercises 9 minutes	Cardio (Power Intervals) 4 intervals 18 minutes
2	Resistance (Muscle Balancing) 1 circuit 9 exercises 9 minutes	Cardio (Speed Intervals) 5 intervals 17 minutes	Resistance (Muscle Balancing) 1 circuit 9 exercises 9 minutes	Cardio (1-Minute Intervals) 5 intervals 19 minutes	Resistance (Muscle Balancing) 1 circuit 9 exercises 9 minutes	Cardio (Power Intervals) 5 intervals 21 minutes
3	Resistance (Muscle Balancing) 2 circuits 9 exercises 18 minutes	Cardio (Speed Intervals) 6 intervals 18 minutes	Resistance (Muscle Balancing) 2 circuits 9 exercises 18 minutes	Cardio (1-Minute Intervals) 6 intervals 21 minutes	Resistance (Muscle Balancing) 2 circuits 9 exercises 18 minutes	Cardio (Power Intervals) 6 intervals 23 minutes
4	Resistance (Muscle Balancing) 1 circuit 9 exercises 9 minutes	Cardio (Speed Intervals) 4 intervals 15 minutes	Resistance (Muscle Balancing) 1 circuit 9 exercises 9 minutes	Cardio (1-Minute Intervals) 4 intervals 17 minutes	Resistance (Muscle Balancing) 1 circuit 9 exercises 9 minutes	Cardio (Power Intervals) 4 intervals 18 minutes

ADVANCED SCHEDULE

Wk #	Monday	Tuesday	Wednesday	Thursday	Friday	Saturday
1	Resistance (Muscle Balancing) 1 circuit 12 exercises 12 minutes	Cardio (Speed Intervals) 6 intervals 18 minutes	Resistance (Muscle Balancing) 1 circuit 12 exercises 12 minutes	Cardio (1-Minute Intervals) 6 intervals 21 minutes	Resistance (Muscle Balancing) 1 circuit 12 exercises 12 minutes	Cardio (Power Intervals) 6 intervals 23 minutes
2	Resistance (Muscle Balancing) 1 circuit 12 exercises 12 minutes	Cardio (Speed Intervals) 7 intervals 20 minutes	Resistance (Muscle Balancing) 1 circuit 12 exercises 12 minutes	Cardio (1-Minute Intervals) 7 intervals 23 minutes	Resistance (Muscle Balancing) 1 circuit 12 exercises 12 minutes	Cardio (Power Intervals) 7 intervals 26 minutes
3	Resistance (Muscle Balancing) 2 circuits 12 exercises 24 minutes	Cardio (Speed Intervals) 8 intervals 21 minutes	Resistance (Muscle Balancing) 2 circuits 12 exercises 24 minutes	Cardio (1-Minute Intervals) 8 intervals 25 minutes	Resistance (Muscle Balancing) 2 circuits 12 exercises 24 minutes	Cardio (Power Intervals) 8 intervals 28 minutes
4	Resistance (Muscle Balancing) 1 circuit 12 exercises 12 minutes	Cardio (Speed Intervals) 6 intervals 18 minutes	Resistance (Muscle Balancing) 1 circuit 12 exercises 12 minutes	Cardio (1-Minute Intervals) 6 intervals 21 minutes	Resistance (Muscle Balancing) 1 circuit 12 exercises 12 minutes	Cardio (Power Intervals) 6 intervals 23 minutes

CHAPTER 5

Nutrition:

Key Food

Substitutions

If you're like most men and women who are unhappy about the amount of fat on their bodies, you view your appetite as an enemy. Excessive appetite causes you to eat more food than you need each day, and as a result you gain fat. If you try to eat any less than your appetite demands, hunger nags you until you give in and resume obeying your appetite.

It's not really fair to blame your appetite for your body fat level, however. The human appetite is in fact a highly tuned and precisely regulated mechanism that has been calibrated through eons of evolution to ensure that you eat just the right amount of food to meet your needs. Unfortunately our living environment has changed in two significant ways since nature put the finishing touches on our appetite.

First, our lifestyle has become much more sedentary than it used to be. Our appetite was designed to make us eat enough food to stay lean, strong, and healthy at a high level of daily activity. When we become inactive, as most of us are today, our appetite decreases very little, if at all, so we continue to eat just as much food and store the excess calories as body fat.

In addition, our food supply has changed drastically within the past century or so. We now eat more foods that are calorically dense, meaning they pack a lot of calories in a small amount of food volume. Processed foods containing large amounts of fat and carbohydrate—such as french fries and candy bars—are especially calorically dense. At the same time, we are eating far fewer foods that are less calorically dense—fruits and vegetables in particular. Research has shown that our appetite is designed to make us eat a certain volume of food each day, regardless of the number of calories contained in that total food volume. When our diet is based on the natural, noncalorically dense foods our ancestors ate, the volume of food that satisfies our appetite supplies just enough calories to keep us lean, strong, and healthy. But when our diet is based on calorically dense processed foods, as it is for most of us today, the volume of food that satisfies our appetite provides more calories than we need, and as a result we store fat.

The good news is that even today you can still trust your appetite to tell you the right amount of food to eat to become leaner, stronger, and healthier. And you can do this without forcing yourself to eat less food than you need to feel satisfied. All you have to do is increase your activity level and make some key substitutions in your diet that reduce the number of calories you consume without reducing the volume of food you eat.

THE SUBSTITUTION STRATEGY

In my work as a dietician I never ask my clients to eat less. Instead I always suggest the following food substitutions to help them cut calories without reducing the volume of food they consume:

1. Replace a nonvegetable food with a vegetable (or increase a vegetable portion).
2. Replace a nonfruit food with a fruit (or increase a fruit portion).

3. Replace a high-calorie beverage with a low-calorie beverage.
4. Replace a fried food with a nonfried food.
5. Replace a high-fat meat with a lean meat.
6. Replace a high-calorie sauce, condiment, or topping with a low-calorie alternative.
7. Replace a refined grain with a whole grain.
8. Replace a whole-milk dairy food with a low-fat dairy food.
9. Replace a high-calorie dessert with a low-calorie dessert.
10. Replace a nonorganic food with an organic food.

You will find that introducing each of these changes into your diet is a lot easier than going on a conventional weight-loss program, because each change is small and easy to make, yet the combination of all ten makes a big impact. It's important to note that these substitutions do not represent a short-term weight-loss diet; they represent permanent changes to your eating habits that will help you get lean quickly and stay lean for life.

Here's how to kick-start your new eating habits. First, make a list of the foods you typically eat for all of your meals and snacks. Next, match this list against the ten key substitutions to identify specific opportunities to make calorie-cutting substitutions to the staple foods in your diet. Begin to implement your substitutions on the first day of the Lean Look program, and never go back to the way you used to eat.

Of course, you won't always eat the same way every day, but you will find that it's very easy to transfer particular substitutions to any other meal or snack. For example, suppose you normally eat a sandwich for lunch, and you choose to cut calories by replacing your plain roast-beef sandwich with a veggie-packed sandwich wrap (an example of substitution #1). But perhaps you occasionally like to break routine by going out for Chinese food with coworkers at lunchtime. You can easily transfer your lunch substitution to this meal by choosing an entrée with vegetables and eating it without rice. It's just another way to practice substitution #1.

Make your best effort to take advantage of every opportunity to make a calorie-cutting substitution, but don't worry about the occasional missed opportunity or lapse. As long as you practice most of the substitutions most of the time, you will consistently consume the right number of calories to get leaner and then stay lean. And there's no need to count the number of calories you eat or aim to cut a certain number of calories from your "normal" diet. One of the major advantages of the key substitutions strategy is that it spares you the hassle of calorie counting by enabling you to trust your appetite to regulate your calorie intake automatically.

See Appendix B for a complete four-week meal plan based on these ten key substitutions. You are invited to rely on this meal plan for your Phase I nutrition as an easy way to get accustomed to lean eating. By the time you complete this four-week meal plan you will have enough experience in lean eating to confidently guide your own substitutions in the future.

The meal plan does not provide suggested portion sizes because you can rely on your appetite to appropriately regulate the amount of food you eat. Just prepare and eat enough to feel satisfied by each meal and snack. The caloric density of the foods in this meal plan is so low that you would have to eat to the point of uncomfortable fullness to spoil your effort to get lean.

Note that the meal plan does not integrate the nutrient timing practices that constitute the nutrition component of Phase II. In chapter 9 I will show you how to easily modify the eating plan to incorporate nutrient timing.

THE TEN KEY CALORIE-CUTTING FOOD SUBSTITUTIONS

Now let's take a detailed look at each of the ten key calorie-cutting food substitutions that you will introduce into your diet.

SUBSTITUTION #1: REPLACE A NONVEGETABLE FOOD WITH A VEGETABLE.

Besides being packed with vitamins, minerals, and phytonutrients (nourishing plant chemicals), most vegetables also contain lots of fiber and water. Why is this important? As I have said earlier, research has shown that we tend to eat a consistent volume of food each day, regardless of how many calories are contained in it. Water and fiber increase the volume of foods without increasing calories. Vegetables are said to be less "calorically dense" than other foods because their high water and fiber content makes them fill a large volume of space in your stomach compared to other foods of equal calories. For example, cooked zucchini contains just 16 calories per 100 grams, whereas Cheddar cheese contains 100 calories per 100 grams. Therefore by replacing any nonvegetable food in your diet (e.g., meats, grains, dairy products) with a vegetable, you can cut calories without actually eating less. It really doesn't matter what kind of nonvegetable food you replace with a vegetable, because vegetables are less calorically dense than every other kind of food. (The only exception is fresh fruit. I don't recommend swapping fruits with vegetables because they are equally important for leanness and good health.)

The effectiveness of food substitutions was demonstrated in a Penn State study in which women were fed either a high-density, medium-density, or low-density meal three times a day. All participants received instructions to eat as much as they wanted. The subjects in all three groups ate the same weight of food, but the women eating the high-density meals took in 30 percent more calories than the women eating the low-density meals owing to the differences in caloric density.

The lunch entrée, for example, was a pasta bake made from pasta shells, zucchini, broccoli, carrots, onions, tomato sauce, and Parmesan, mozzarella, and ricotta cheeses. The low-density version contained more vegetables, while the medium- and high-density versions contained more shells and cheese. This example demonstrates how you can reduce your daily caloric intake in general without "eating less," and without necessarily eating different foods. Merely changing the proportions can do the trick!

Replace french fries with a salad.

A simple substitution that I recommend to my clients who sometimes eat at fast food restaurants is to order a side salad instead of french fries. Most of the major chains have recently made this substitution easier and more affordable by allowing customers to choose a side salad as part of their regular "combo" deals. It's amazing how long it took McDonald's and their competitors to think of offering this simple option, but hey, better late than never.

Eat a double portion of cooked vegetables with dinner.

I have found that the simplest way to cut the number of calories you eat during meals is to serve yourself a larger portion of vegetables and smaller portions of the other foods in the meal. Suppose you're having broiled salmon, a large serving (1 cup) of mashed potatoes, and a small garden salad for dinner. By cutting the size of your mashed potatoes serving in half and doubling the size of your salad, you'll cut nearly 100 calories from this meal. The meal remains essentially the same; only the proportions change.

Add more vegetables to pasta dishes, stir-fries, and other dishes.

Here are other examples of ways to make this substitution:

- Make a stir-fry with more vegetables and less meat and/or rice.
- Have a burrito with less meat and more beans and grilled veggies added.
- Eat kebabs with less meat and more veggies.
- Choose a pizza with a thinner crust, slightly less cheese, and vegetable toppings (e.g., tomatoes and green peppers).

You don't have to follow any strict formula, but as a general guideline, try to increase the size of your vegetable portion by 50–100 percent.

If you are not currently eating any vegetables with your meals (except perhaps pickles and onions on your hamburgers!), you will need to begin by simply adding real vegetables to your meals. Just add a salad or a cooked vegetable to your lunch or dinner and "make room" for it by eating slightly less meat, less grains, or less of whatever else you're having.

The USDA recommends that adult women eat approximately $2\frac{1}{2}$ cups of cooked vegetables per day. Men should aim for 3 cups. (Note that salads count for only $\frac{1}{2}$ cup per 1 cup you eat because they are much less dense than cooked veggies.) You may need to make more than one vegetable substitution to reach this recommendation. That's okay—don't feel compelled to get there in one giant leap. Each substitution will trim substantial calories from your diet and move you closer to the Lean Look.

If you've somehow convinced yourself that you don't like vegetables, recognize that there are hundreds of different vegetables and thousands of ways to prepare them. You're bound to like at least a few forms of vegetables. Baked beans count as a vegetable. The romaine lettuce in a grilled chicken Caesar salad counts. Even a bowl of tomato soup counts as a vegetable serving. Put a little thought and effort into drawing up a list of vegetable dishes you do like and don't feel guilty about eating these dishes and ignoring the ones you don't like. (As time goes by you will probably find that your list of acceptable vegetable dishes grows and grows.) There are five basic categories of vegetables, and it's a good idea to hit all of them on a regular basis, as each has a nutrient profile that's different from the others. The five categories are dark green, orange, legumes, starchy, and other vegetables. Here are examples of each:

DARK GREEN	ORANGE	LEGUMES	STARCHY	OTHER
Bok choy	Acorn squash	Black beans	Corn	Artichokes
Broccoli	Butternut squash	Black-eyed peas	Green peas	Asparagus
Collard greens	Carrots	Garbanzo beans (chickpeas)	Potatoes	Beets
Dark green leafy lettuce	Pumpkin	Kidney beans		Brussels sprouts
Kale	Sweet potatoes	Lentils		Cabbage
Mustard greens		Lima beans		Cauliflower
Romaine lettuce		Navy beans		Cucumbers
Spinach		Pinto beans		Eggplant
Turnip greens		Soybeans		Green beans
Watercress		Split peas		Okra
		White beans		Onions
				Sweet peppers
				Tomatoes
				Vegetable juice
				Zucchini

SUBSTITUTION #2: REPLACE A NONFRUIT FOOD WITH A FRUIT.

Like vegetables, most fruits are high in water and fiber content, so they fill you up with fewer calories. There are three good ways to make fruit substitutions in your diet.

Add fruits to meals.

One option is to add fruits to foods or meals and reduce the amount of the other food(s) you're eating. For example, instead of eating a whole 8-ounce tub of yogurt (232 calories), eat a bowl of berries (½ cup) drizzled with non-fat vanilla yogurt (91 calories).

Eat fruit instead of your usual snacks.

A second option is to replace your usual snack foods with fruits. A 1-cup portion of Cheez-Its crackers contains 312 calories. A pear contains just 100 calories. If giving up your usual snack foods completely is too great a hardship, you can eat smaller portions of them along with fruit and still come out ahead calorically. If you eat ½ cup of Cheez-Its (156 calories) and a small pear (85 calories), you'll consume a total of 241 calories—still 51 fewer calories than are contained in a full cup of Cheez-Its.

Have fruit-based desserts.

Since many fruits taste sweet, they make excellent desserts. In fact, I consider fruits to be nature's desserts! You can trim a lot of calories by incorporating fruits into your desserts. A slice of homemade apple pie has 265 calories, compared to 367 calories in a slice of frosted chocolate cake. Some other examples of low-calorie fruit-based desserts are fresh mixed berries with light whipped cream, peach cobbler, caramelized bananas, and mango sticky rice.

Men and women alike should aim to consume at least 2 cups of fruit per day. Fresh, canned, frozen, dried, cut, and puréed fruits all count toward this total, as do 100 percent fruit juices (although these lack the fiber that is in solid fruit). As you do with vegetables, try to eat a variety of different fruits. There are dozens of delicious options, ranging from berries to citrus fruits such as tangerines and grapefruit to autumn fruits including apples and pears. Eat your favorites and leave those you aren't crazy about for someone else.

SUBSTITUTION #3: REPLACE A HIGH-CALORIE BEVERAGE WITH A LOW-CALORIE BEVERAGE.

One of the easiest ways to trim a surprising number of calories from your daily intake is to make a few key beverage substitutions. America has become a beverage-crazy society during my lifetime, and I believe this trend has had a significant impact on our bodies. The sheer variety of beverages available in stores has exploded, and serving sizes have also increased substantially. Currently one in five calories in the average American's diet comes from beverages.

By reversing this trend with some key substitutions you can also reverse its effects on your body. This was demonstrated by a study done at Children's Hospital in Boston. Researchers there invited 103 teens to pick noncaloric drinks they liked and then delivered a supply of those drinks to their home refrigerators. Consumption of sugar-sweetened beverages tumbled by 82 percent over a six-month period, the researchers reported. The subjects also lost 1 pound of body weight per month on average in the study period.

One of my early clients, Wayne, drank six to eight sodas a day when he started working with me. Not surprisingly, he was overweight and had high blood sugar, high blood pressure, elevated bad cholesterol and low good cholesterol, and other health problems ranging from poor sleep to chronic constipation. I had Wayne gradually replace his sodas with bottled water, one by one, until he was down to just a few sodas a week. The only other dietary change I prescribed was an increase in his fruit and vegetable consumption, from zero servings up to four to eight servings per day. He also started working out three to four times a week. Within forty days Wayne had lost 13 pounds, and eventually he lost 16 pounds more and achieved a 32 percent body fat reduction. His blood pressure, blood sugar, and bad cholesterol dropped significantly, while his good cholesterol rose. His health complaints went away and he felt better all around. Those are big results from rather modest lifestyle changes!

There are three basic categories of beverages that hide a lot of calories: caffeinated beverages, soft drinks, and alcoholic drinks.

Replace high-calorie caffeine drinks with lower-calorie alternatives.

Plain tea and coffee contain minimal calories, but the sugar- and fat-filled drinks that are frequently made with coffee and tea have plenty. A Venti (large) Caffé Latte from Starbucks contains a whopping 340 calories. By replacing the whole milk it contains with nonfat milk you will reduce the calories to 210. By ordering a Grande (medium) size instead you'll lop off another

50 calories. Or you could just get a good old-fashioned small coffee, sweeten it with half-and-half and a sugar packet, and get your caffeine fix with just 41 calories. If you currently consume large servings of caffeinated drinks with a lot of additives, make these substitutions and prepare to reap the benefits.

Most health-conscious individuals who have a major caffeine habit already order "light" versions of their drinks, but don't kid yourself—these drinks still have a lot of calories. For example, a Grande Starbucks Caffè Vanilla Frappuccino Light with no whipped cream contains 230 calories. Treating yourself to one such drink in the morning and one in the evening is tantamount to eating a second lunch. No matter how "light" you make your caffeinated beverages, you should limit yourself to no more than one 16-ounce serving per day, because the calories add up and too much caffeine isn't good for you anyway.

One of my clients, Greg, came to me because he had mysteriously begun to add belly fat in recent months despite the fact that his overall diet was very healthy and he worked out regularly. When I analyzed Greg's diet I discovered that he was consuming an enormous number of calories in his morning latte. I showed him how to cut back on these calories and once he did he quickly lost that belly fat.

Replace sugary drinks with sugar-free drinks.

Sodas such as Coca-Cola contribute more calories to the average American's diet than any other single "food" source. A 12-ounce can of Coca-Cola contains 140 calories. It also contains virtually no nutrition, so these calories are pure, useless excess. The same is true of other sugary beverages ranging from lemonade to "energy" drinks such as Red Bull. My first recommendation is that you replace all such drinks in your diet, except for the occasional treat, with water, which has 0 calories. If you must have something sweet, choose low- or no-calorie alternatives to sugary beverages such as flavored water or diet soda. I have some reservations about recommending diet soft drinks because research has shown that those who consume them regularly are more likely to become overweight than those who don't, possibly because the knowledge that these drinks are low calorie makes people feel free to load up on food calories. But I still think a 0-calorie soda is better than a 140-calorie soda, provided you switch to the former as part of a general effort to trim excess calories from your diet.

Replace alcoholic beverages with light alternatives.
Alcoholic beverages are another source of useless calories. Limit yourself to one or at most two alcoholic drinks per day. If you drink beer, consider switching your regular beer for a light beer—by doing so you'll trim roughly 60 calories. After that first alcoholic drink, for any additional drinks you're tempted to have, substitute a low-calorie "mocktail" such as club soda on ice with a twist of lemon or a dash of cranberry juice.

SUBSTITUTION #4: REPLACE A FRIED FOOD WITH A NONFRIED FOOD.

Oils used for frying add a lot of fat calories to foods that would otherwise be fairly lean. Frying also creates artery-clogging trans fats. Sometimes it's hard to say "no" to fried foods, but it's easier when you can say "yes" to alternatives that are also quite delicious. For example, a serving of Spicy Chicken Strips (breaded and fried) from Popeye's restaurant has 310 calories. A serving of Popeye's Naked Chicken Strips (roasted) has just 170 calories—and they're just as tasty.

Not all frying is bad. There's an important distinction to be made between what I call "heavy frying," which is bad, and "light frying," which is okay. You can be sure that most fried foods you get at restaurants are heavy-fried. Heavy frying includes deep-frying (where the food being cooked is fully immersed in oil) and pan-frying involving large amounts of oil, grease, lard, or butter. Light frying is pan-frying using just enough fat to prevent your food from sticking to the pan or burning. The best fat to use for pan-frying is olive oil. You can make relatively lean stir-fries, pan-fried meats and fish, egg and egg-substitute omelets, hash brown potatoes, and other such foods by using olive oil (which produces few trans fats) sparingly—again, just enough to prevent your food from sticking to the pan or burning.

Just about any heavy-fried food you can imagine has a nonfried alternative that is much lower in calories. Here are three examples.

Replace breaded, deep-fried meat and fish with alternatives.
Instead of eating breaded and fried chicken or fish, eat chicken or fish broiled, baked, steamed, grilled, or poached. Replace your french fries with a baked

potato, or roasted, boiled, or mashed potatoes; a yam; or even a light potato salad.

Replace fried snack chips with alternatives.

There are also many leaner alternatives to common fried snack chips such as potato chips (155 calories per 1-ounce serving) and Doritos (150 calories per ounce). Baked chips (110 calories) are the obvious choice, but other options include popcorn (110 calories), whole-wheat pretzels (103 calories), dried fruit (70 calories per ounce), and baby carrots dipped in ranch dressing (33 calories per ounce).

Replace other fried foods with alternatives.

Among the many other fried foods for which you should find substitutes except on special occasions are donuts (try a low-fat muffin instead), egg rolls (go for a fresh spring roll), and enchiladas (swap them for soft tacos).

SUBSTITUTION #5: REPLACE A HIGH-FAT MEAT WITH A LEAN MEAT.

Some meats have a lot more fat than others. Those with the least fat have the fewest calories. Make every effort to substitute leaner meats for the fatty meats you're eating. It's easy.

Replace fatty cuts of any type of meat with leaner cuts of the same type.

For example, by replacing an 85-percent lean ground beef hamburger patty with a 95-percent lean ground beef hamburger patty you'll take in 60 fewer calories. You're still eating ground beef, but it's leaner, and will therefore help you get leaner, too.

Check out the following chart for a list of fatty meats that should be swapped out of your diet and a list of the lean meats that should be brought in to replace them. All fish is acceptable except for tuna packed in oil. (By eating a 6-ounce can of tuna packed in water instead of one packed in oil, you'll consume 190 calories instead of 340.)

FATTY MEATS	LEAN MEATS
Bacon	Beef tenderloin
Bologna	Canned tuna (water packed)
Canned tuna (packed in oil)	Chicken breasts (boneless, skinless)
Chicken with skin	
Eggs	Egg substitutes
Ground beef (regular)	Fish
Ground turkey (regular	Ground beef (extra lean)
Ham	Ground turkey (extra lean)
Lamb	London broil
Prime cut beef	Organic meats (grass-fed)
Pork chop	Pork tenderloin (lean)
Rib-eye steak	Roast beef
Salami	Turkey breast
Sausage	
T-bone steak	
Veal	

Replace whole eggs with egg whites.
While eggs technically are not a meat, I include them in the list of fatty meats, and egg substitutes (i.e., egg whites) on the list of lean meats. Whole eggs are fine in moderation, but if you eat eggs regularly, be sure to substitute egg whites for some of them.

Replace red meat with poultry and poultry with fish.
Fish has fewer calories per ounce than chicken, chicken has fewer than turkey, and turkey has fewer than red meat. So, in addition to eating leaner versions of each type of meat (e.g., trading your T-bone steak for a London broil), it's a good idea to shift the balance of your meat intake away from red meat and toward fish and poultry.

SUBSTITUTION #6: REPLACE A HIGH-CALORIE SAUCE, CONDIMENT, OR TOPPING WITH A LOW-CALORIE ALTERNATIVE.

Sauces, condiments, and toppings are another sneaky source of extra calories in the average person's diet. You might be amazed to learn how many calories some of these foods have, and how many calories you can easily trim from your diet by using lighter substitutions. (See chart below for some examples.)

There are three specific ways to practice this substitution strategy.

Replace a high-calorie sauce, condiment, or topping with a light version of the same.
Substitute the sauces, condiments, and toppings you normally use with reduced-calorie versions of the same. There are light versions of almost everything, including mayonnaise, salad dressings, and peanut butter. Each one alone will not cut a ton of calories from your diet, but if you choose these products at every opportunity, the savings in calories will really add up, as you can see in the chart below.

CALORIE COMPARISONS BETWEEN REGULAR AND LOWER-CALORIE VERSIONS OF SAUCES, CONDIMENTS, AND TOPPINGS

Regular mayonnaise	57 calories per tablespoon
Light mayonnaise	32 calories per tablespoon
Regular Italian salad dressing	43 calories per tablespoon
Fat-free Italian salad dressing	7 calories per tablespoon
Regular peanut butter	94 calories per tablespoon
Reduced-fat peanut butter	83 calories per tablespoon
Regular barbecue sauce	45 calories per serving
Walden Farms calorie free original barbecue sauce	0 calories per serving
Strawberry jam	50 calories per tablespoon
100% fruit strawberry preserves	40 calories per tablespoon

Replace a high-calorie sauce, condiment, or topping with a lower-calorie alternative.

You can often trim even more calories by replacing high-calorie sauces, condiments, and toppings not with lighter versions of the same things but instead with completely different alternatives. For example, if you normally use mayonnaise (57 calories) on your sandwiches, use mustard (14 calories) instead. Rather than putting butter (100 calories) on your baked potato, drizzle a little vinegar (3 calories) over it or sprinkle it with Parmesan cheese (30 calories). Use a salsa (33 calories) to flavor your poultry and fish dishes instead of heavy sauces such as a cream sauce (92 calories).

Reduce the amount of any given sauce, condiment, or topping you use.

Simply cutting back on the amount of sauces, condiments, and toppings you use is also a viable strategy in the case of this particular substitution, because we really don't rely on these foods to satisfy our hunger. They merely provide flavor. Try to use no more than half the amount of sauces, condiments, and toppings you would normally use. Put just enough (reduced-fat) mayonnaise in your tuna salad to hold it together. Use a very light coating of barbecue sauce on your chicken. Toss your salads with as little dressing as necessary to give them flavor. Eat unfrosted or unglazed cakes instead of heavily frosted ones. You get the idea.

SUBSTITUTION #7: REPLACE A REFINED GRAIN WITH A WHOLE GRAIN.

Processed grains such as white flour and white rice have been stripped of their natural fiber content (as well as most of their vitamins and minerals), making them a lot more calorically dense than whole-grain foods such as whole wheat flour and brown rice. Switching from processed grains to whole grains is a very simple and nondisruptive way to shave some calories off your daily intake while adding fiber to your diet.

Replace white rice with brown rice and regular pasta with whole-wheat pasta.

For many of us, rice and pasta are meal staples that make an appearance on our dinner plate a couple of times per week or more. Forget about the low-carb diets that tell you not to eat these foods. Instead trim calories by replacing white rice with brown rice and regular white flour pasta with whole-wheat pasta. By replacing a cup of cooked white rice with a cup of brown rice you save 26 calories. A cup of cooked regular spaghetti noodles contains 221 calories, compared to just 174 in a cup of cooked whole-wheat pasta.

Replace processed-grain breads with 100 percent whole-grain breads.

Breads made with whole grains are also less calorically dense than breads made with refined versions of the same grains. Eat a sandwich made with whole-wheat bread instead of white bread and save 22 calories. Read labels to make sure the products you buy are made entirely with whole grains. Some products whose packaging boasts that they are "made with whole grains" contain both whole grain and processed grain.

Replace high-sugar breakfast cereals with lower-sugar breakfast cereals.

Consider sugar a processed grain and do your best to avoid it, too. Table sugar, or sucrose, is derived from sugarcane and sugar beets through a process that is similar to the process used to create refined flour, and with similar results. At more than 4 calories per gram, table sugar is one of the most calorically dense foods in existence. Corn syrup, derived from corn, is another one to watch out for. These sugars are added in copious amounts to all kinds of products that don't really need them, from breakfast cereals and breads to salad dressings and steak sauces. Again, read labels and choose products that contain little or no added sugar. You'll trim substantial calories by making this small effort. To give just one example, Apple Jacks breakfast cereal is made with refined grains and contains 16 grams of sugar and 130 calories per serving. Whole-grain Cheerios breakfast cereal contains just 1.2 grams of sugar and 110 calories per serving.

SUBSTITUTION #8: REPLACE A WHOLE-MILK DAIRY FOOD WITH A LOW-FAT DAIRY FOOD.

Most Americans eat more fat than they should and far too much saturated fat. About 15 percent of the calories in the typical American diet come from saturated fat. Nutrition scientists recommend that we get less than 10 percent of our calories from saturated fat. Whole milk and dairy foods made with whole milk contain a lot of fat and a lot of saturated fat, so substitutes should be used whenever possible.

Use skim milk instead of whole milk for drinking, in breakfast cereal, coffee, and so forth.
An easy way to cut back on fat calories and saturated fat intake—not to mention total calories in your diet—is to use skim milk instead of whole milk at every opportunity. Eight ounces of whole milk contain 146 calories. An equal amount of skim milk has just 83 calories. Use skim milk instead of whole milk in your breakfast cereal. If you like coffee with your cereal, and you like milk in your coffee, use skim milk in your coffee, too. And if you're cooking or baking using a recipe that calls for milk, use skim then as well.

Replace yogurt, cheeses, and other dairy foods made from whole milk with alternatives made with skim milk.
There are reduced-fat and nonfat versions of every type of dairy product, including milk, cream, sandwich cheese, pizza cheese, taco cheese, yogurt, frozen yogurt, and ice cream.

Men and women alike are advised to consume three servings of dairy per day. (A serving is 8 ounces of milk or yogurt or 2 ounces of cheese.) By getting each of these servings from low-fat sources you will save quite a few calories over the course of an entire week.

SUBSTITUTION #9: REPLACE A HIGH-CALORIE DESSERT WITH A LOW-CALORIE DESSERT.

Some people don't have a sweet tooth, don't crave desserts, and seldom eat them. If you are such a person, more power to you. Don't change. If you do have a sweet tooth and you just don't consider your dinner complete until you've followed it with something sweet, then substitute low-calorie alternatives for the high-calorie desserts you now eat.

Replace any dessert with a fruit-based dessert.
As I mentioned earlier, fruit-based desserts tend to be lower in calories than most other desserts. A small bowl (½ cup) of ice cream has 143 calories. A large serving (1 cup) of mixed berries with a heaping tablespoon of low-fat vanilla yogurt drizzled on top contains exactly half as many calories.

Replace any dessert with dark chocolate.
Another dessert substitute that I frequently recommend is dark chocolate, for two reasons. Dark chocolate releases mood-boosting chemicals in the brain, so just a single 50-calorie piece can satisfy you better than a whole bowl of sorbet. In addition, dark chocolate is rich in antioxidants that are good for the heart. Dark chocolate is calorically dense, however, so it's important that you limit yourself to just one small piece. But again, dark chocolate is so uniquely satisfying that if you're like me one small piece will fully satisfy your sweet tooth.

Replace any dessert with a gelatin-based dessert.
A third type of dessert substitution that will reduce calories is gelatin-based desserts. Gelatin is a protein product derived from animal collagen and has very low caloric density. Gelatin-based sweets include Jell-O (83 calories per ½ cup), jelly beans (105 calories per ounce), and gummy bears (108 calories per ounce).

Replace a high-fat dessert with a low-fat dessert.
Many desserts, including ice cream and cookies, are high in both sugar and fat. You can reduce the number of calories you get from these types of desserts by eating low-fat and nonfat versions of them. For example, a slice of fat-free pound

cake has roughly 28 fewer calories than a slice of regular pound cake. Sure, fat-free pound cake still has a lot of sugar in it, but the point of the key substitutions strategy is not to make your diet perfect but to improve your existing eating habits. So, if chocolate chip cookies have a place in your current diet, then replacing them with low-fat chocolate chip cookies will be beneficial to you.

SUBSTITUTION #10: REPLACE A NONORGANIC FOOD WITH AN ORGANIC FOOD.

Organic foods are plant and animal foods produced in somewhat old-fashioned ways that forsake some of the modern technological shortcuts that make our food less healthy. Organic fruits and vegetables are produced without the use of chemical agents (pesticides, fungicides, etc.) and usually grow in much richer soil than do nonorganic plant foods (soil with more minerals and only natural fertilizers). Numerous studies have shown that the nutrient-poor soil in which most nonorganic plants are grown yields fruits and vegetables with lesser amounts of vitamins, minerals, and phytonutrients. Organic plant foods are not lower in calories than their nonorganic counterparts, but they do provide more nutrition per calorie, so they're always a better choice. There are two other ways to replace nonorganic foods with organic alternatives and often cut calories at the same time.

Replace nonorganic meats and farm-raised fish with organic meats and wild fish.

Organic animal foods (meat and fish) are leaner than nonorganic ones owing to the freedom of movement the animals enjoy during their lifetime and their superior diet. For example, organic chicken contains about a third less fat than nonorganic chicken. Wild salmon has more than 25 percent less fat than farm-raised salmon. And a 6-ounce beef loin from a grass-fed cow contains roughly 92 fewer calories than a 6-ounce loin from a grain-fed cow.

Replace regular packaged foods with organic packaged foods.

You can also buy organic versions of boxed and canned foods and other packaged foods. In addition to containing organically produced ingredients, such products do not contain most of the unhealthy additives (artificial colorings, preservatives, etc.) that are common in their nonorganic counterparts. Organic packaged products are typically made with fewer and better-quality ingredients, and as a result they are frequently lower in calories. For example, a serving of Walnut Acres Organic Four Bean Chili contains 140 calories, or 60 fewer calories than an equal serving of nonorganic Stagg Vegetable Garden Four-Bean Chili.

Organic foods are more expensive and in many cases harder to come by than nonorganic foods, and they aren't always lower in calories. But they are always more nutritious, and more often than not you do save calories when you substitute an organic food for a nonorganic one, so I recommend that you make this type of substitution whenever it's convenient.

TAKING THE LONG VIEW

The key substitutions strategy is all about effecting small changes that add up. By making simple substitutions to your current meals and snacks at every opportunity—you will cut a few calories here and a few there until you reach a total calorie reduction that is adequate to strip excess fat stores from your body. And again, there is no need to aim for any specific daily calorie intake or calorie-cutting total. Making the ten key substitutions will give your appetite the opportunity to determine the right amount of food to eat, especially when you combine this strategy with the nutrient timing strategies that you will integrate into your diet in Phase II and your Lean Look resistance and cardio workouts.

Keep in mind that the key substitution strategy is not a short-term diet but a permanent lifestyle change, so it's important to make changes you can live with for the long haul. For this reason you may even wish to add new substitutions gradually, rather than trying to make them all at once and risking burnout.

In any case, it will surely take some time to truly master the key substitutions strategy. For example, if you prepare most of your dinners and you seldom include vegetables, you will probably have to expand your repertoire of vegetable dishes before you're able to fully execute substitution #1. It might also take some time to change your shopping habits—to find suitable substitutes for many of the products you currently buy. Be patient with this process. Most substitutions are simple enough to implement quickly, but as an overall strategy the ten key substitutions will surely get you going on a learning curve, and that's a good thing. It's up to you to find the specific substitutions within each type that fit your tastes, preferences, and lifestyle. This process will probably never cease. In a few years you will be familiar with dozens more ways to make calorie-cutting substitutions.

The only way to be certain that a substitute food has fewer calories than the food it is replacing is, of course, to know how many calories are in each. In many cases it will be perfectly obvious, as when you replace a bowl of ice cream with a single, small piece of dark chocolate. But your efforts to make good substitutions will get a boost if you have numbers in front of you. All packaged foods have labels that provide these numbers. Just compare the calories per serving in one versus the calories per serving in the other (and make sure the serving sizes match up). You can also purchase a book with nutrition information for hundreds of foods, such as *The Complete Book of Food Counts* by Corinne T. Netzer. In addition, many Web sites provide this information (e.g., www.calorielab.com).

CHAPTER 6

Resistance Exercise: Muscle Balancing

Mike is a business executive in his forties who came to me for help in breaking out of a fitness rut. Despite working out six days a week, he was having no success in achieving his goal of adding muscle mass while keeping his overall body weight the same. After firing questions at Mike for just a few minutes I knew exactly why. Mike had been doing the same workouts for twenty years. There was no variation, no progression, no step-by-step sequence leading Mike from where he was to where he wanted to be. As I always tell my clients, "If your workouts don't change, you won't either."

I showed Mike how to create a periodized long-term training plan with separate phases. In each new phase he would do workouts in a slightly different way than he had in the preceding phase. The new training emphasis in each phase would challenge his muscles to develop beyond the level they had already. The workouts would be carefully ordered so that the gains he made in the current phase prepared him for the new challenges presented by the next. Within a few weeks of starting the program I designed for him Mike reported to me that he had busted through his fitness plateau and was gaining muscle size and strength for the first time in years.

As this example illustrates, when you're trying to develop any type of skill or aptitude, it's important to do things in the proper order. For example, if you want to become a mathematician, you'd better learn basic algebra before you tackle advanced calculus, because you can do basic algebra without knowing advanced calculus, but you can't do advanced calculus without knowing basic algebra.

The same principle applies to resistance exercise. There are several different ways to develop muscle tone and there's a proper order in which to do them. The specific type of resistance exercise that is fundamental to all of the others, and must therefore precede the others, is muscle balancing, or what we strength and conditioning coaches call *anatomical adaptation* or *prehabilitation*. The purpose of muscle-balancing exercises is to prepare your muscles to take on more challenging muscle-development exercises later. When you begin the muscle-development process, you need to gradually habituate your tendons and other connective tissues to the stress of bearing and pulling against great resistance. You must also teach your brain and muscles to "talk" to each other more efficiently—that is, to enhance what is known as *neuromuscular coordination*. And, finally, you have to begin the process of increasing the strength of your many muscles, especially those muscles that are weakest compared to the others (this is where the notion of "balancing" comes in). Creating a balance of strength among all of your major muscle groups is critical to getting the most out of the more challenging resistance workouts you'll do later, in Phases II and III of the Lean Look program.

The key to getting off to a good start in the muscle-conditioning process is challenging your muscles enough to generate these anatomical adaptations without taking on too much too soon. At this point you need to avoid lifting extremely heavy loads, performing high-speed lifts, doing multi-joint movements that require a bunch of muscle groups to cooperate, and doing exercises that tend to throw you off balance. Instead you want to begin by doing simple, straightforward movements designed to strengthen individual muscle groups in relative isolation from one another, using moderate resistance.

This is the case even if you have past experience with strength training. A good resistance exercise program always starts with a solid foundation, works toward a peak, and then starts over with a new period of foundation building after a short recovery phase. You can't just continue building your muscles indefinitely without interruption. You'll always get the best results in the long run if you train in repeating cycles. No matter how naturally strong you are or how experienced in the gym, you will never outgrow the need to return to foundation building periodically.

The resistance exercises you do in Phase I are for foundation building. You will benefit from these exercises regardless of your strength-training background or current level of muscular fitness. Naturally you will do the workouts in this phase at a different level if you are already able to haul refrigerators on your back than if you have trouble carrying a gallon of milk to your refrigerator from the trunk of your car. But your workouts will share the same basic design and purpose in either case.

Before you begin the Lean Look program, decide whether you will follow the beginner or the advanced workout schedule. Both beginner muscle-balancing resistance workouts and advanced muscle-balancing resistance workouts draw on the same pool of exercises presented in this chapter; advanced workouts just include more of them.

BEFORE YOU BEGIN

There are four important matters to address before we dive into the Phase I muscle-balancing resistance exercises and workouts. First, you need to make sure that you have access to enough equipment to be able to perform complete Lean Look resistance workouts throughout all three phases. Second, I want to show you a quick warm-up that I'd like you to do at the beginning of each resistance workout throughout all three phases. Third, I'll explain how to "set your core" to stabilize and protect your spine when performing all resistance exercises throughout the Lean Look program. And, finally, I will explain something called the "plus-one rule," which will help you select the appropriate resistance level for many exercises.

REQUIRED EQUIPMENT

I've intentionally minimized the amount of equipment required for the resistance exercises in order to make working out at home an affordable option for those who wish to do so. Many of the exercises in all three phases require no equipment. Others require dumbbells, an exercise bench, some form of cable resistance, or a stability ball. You can find a list of popular brands and retailers of all the equipment mentioned here in the "Resources" section at the back of the book (Appendix C).

DUMBBELLS

Dumbbells are the iron in "pumping iron." The smallest ones are half a pound and the largest are—well, let's just say they're heavier than anything you'll ever lift.

The chief advantage of dumbbells is that they are compact and take up little space. Their main drawback is that you need several pairs in order to be able to perform a variety of exercises with appropriate resistance, and they're not as cheap as you might think.

For example, a complete set of dumbbells from 5 to 50 pounds, with a rack, will probably cost you close to $250. Adjustable dumbbells (you buy the handles and weights separately) are cheaper, but require a lot of fuss to change the weight between exercises, making them an especially poor choice for circuit workouts, in which your goal is to minimize time between exercises. The "selectorized" dumbbells, such as PowerBlock and Bowflex SelectTech, are much easier to use and store, but they run several hundred dollars for the basic set and a stand to rest them on.

Your problem is solved if you can work out at a health club, which will have every size of dumbbell.

EXERCISE BENCH

An exercise bench is a flat, padded bench roughly 18 inches high that provides a sturdy platform for various exercises. Some exercise benches feature an adjustable back rest and various attachments, but all you need for the exercises presented here is a nonadjustable flat bench without attachments, which you can get for as little as $50 from an exercise equipment retailer, sporting goods store, or department store. Almost all health clubs are abundantly equipped with such benches.

CABLE RESISTANCE

There are various forms of cable resistance. Whichever one you choose, it must have three things: handles and ankle attachments, high and low attachment points, and adjustable resistance.

The cheapest and most convenient type of cable resistance device for home use is the door gym or wall gym. As the names suggest, these devices mount to a door or wall, providing a secure anchor for exercises involving elastic cable resistance. One example is the Altus door gym, which retails for only $36.99 and offers adjustable resistance levels that enable users of all strength levels to do a wide range of exercises with the right degree of challenge. The Altus door gym uses sturdy bungee cords for resistance and is highly portable; you can easily stuff it in a suitcase and attach it to the door of a hotel room in 30 seconds.

If you move up to roughly the $500 range, you can get a nice wall-mounting unit such as the Lifeline Off-The-Wall gym. Starting at $1,000 are floor-standing home gyms with cable resistance such as the Life Fitness G5. Instead of using elastic resistance, these units use traditional weight stacks. Floor-standing cable-resistance stations offer the advantages of greater adjustability in resistance and superior sturdiness, but in addition to being expensive they are not portable. Most health clubs have cable resistance stations with handle and ankle attachments.

STABILITY BALL

Stability balls are large, inflated plastic balls that you can use in a surprising number of ways in resistance workouts. A high-quality stability ball will cost you $25 to $45. Most fitness clubs have them. Because of their size and the fact that inflating them is a workout in itself, they aren't easy to store or transport. On the bright side, the best ones are durable enough for your kids to play with in between your workouts. Stability balls come in various sizes; be sure to purchase the size that is recommended for your height (this information is usually provided on the packaging). You can purchase a stability ball from exercise equipment and sporting goods retailers.

WARMING UP

Before starting any resistance workout, warm up by completing a few of the following dynamic exercises. These exercises will warm, lubricate, and oxygenate the muscles of your extremities, enhancing their performance in the workout and reducing the likelihood of injury to your muscles and tendons.

DYNAMIC WARM-UP EXERCISES

Do each exercise for 20 seconds.

Ankle flips. Keep your legs straight while hopping up and down on your toes.

Arm circles. Rotate your left arm in a giant circle. Go forward 4 times and backward 4 times. Repeat with your right arm.

Butt kicks. Run in place with your thighs locked in a neutral position and try to kick yourself in the butt with your heels.

High knees. Run in place while lifting your knees as high as you can.

Arm flaps. Raise your arms straight out to the sides. Bring them together and allow them to cross in front of your chest and then flap them back out to the sides.

Squats. Squat down as low as you can comfortably go, and then stand up.

Hip swings. Stand facing a wall and brace your fingers against it for support. Bend forward slightly at the waist. Swing your right leg from side to side in the space between your left leg and the wall. Swing it 8 times and then switch legs.

Frankenstein. Walk forward for 10 steps with your arms extended straight in front of you. Kick your toes up toward your palm with each step. Try to keep your palms even with your toes.

SETTING YOUR CORE

The muscles of the abdominal wall are important stabilizers during all strength exercises. When these muscles are properly activated, there is greater stability in your pelvis and lower spine, which tends to reduce strain on the lower spine and protect it from injury. The problem is that most of us do not activate our core muscles properly when performing strength exercises.

To ensure that you do, practice a technique called "setting your core," or abdominal bracing, before each repetition of every strength exercise. Setting your core consists in simply finding a neutral posture, with your lower spine neither arched nor rounded, and drawing your belly button toward your spine without restricting your breathing or changing the position of your spine. It's a tiny movement, but when you do it you will feel your abdominal muscles tensing and as a result you will feel more "solid" in your midsection. Set your core after assuming the starting position for each exercise but before doing the first repetition. Reset your core during a brief pause after the completion of each repetition. This is necessary because it's all too easy to inadvertently relax the abdominal wall when you stop paying attention to it. Indeed, it's a good idea to concentrate on keeping your abdomen braced throughout each exercise repetition. Eventually setting your core will come more naturally and you won't have to concentrate on it so much.

THE PLUS-ONE RULE

The "plus-one rule" is a guideline that helps you select the appropriate resistance level to use in exercises involving dumbbells and cable resistance and the appropriate number of repetitions to perform in body weight exercises. When applied to dumbbell and cable resistance exercises, the plus-one rule entails choosing a dumbbell weight or cable resistance level that you could lift one more time than you're asked to perform in each "set." You will be asked to complete 12 repetitions of each exercise per set in your muscle-balancing workouts. Thus for each dumbbell and cable resistance exercise you should select a weight/resistance level that you could lift a maximum of 13 times with perfect form. The twelfth and final repetition should be quite challenging, but not so hard that you couldn't squeeze out one more repetition with good form before reaching complete exhaustion.

You will find yourself gaining strength in each exercise over the four weeks of Phase I. Add a repetition to exercises as necessary to maintain a consistent challenge level. Once you're completing 15 repetitions (meaning you're actually able to complete 16), choose a heavier set of dumbbells or increase the level of cable resistance.

When doing body weight exercises, complete one repetition fewer than you could, up to a maximum of 20 repetitions.

MUSCLE-BALANCING RESISTANCE EXERCISES

To do a complete muscle-balancing resistance workout, first complete the warm-up described earlier in this chapter. Having completed your warm-up, perform either 9 or 12 of the muscle-balancing resistance exercises that follow. (Beginner workouts include 9 exercises, while advanced workouts include 12.) Start with a legs exercise, then do a core exercise, and then do an upper body exercise, and continue in this manner until you have completed either 9 exercises or 12. This constitutes one circuit. You can create your own circuits using a combination of the exercises that follow, or you can follow the ready-made circuit workouts provided at the end of the chapter. I also provide a complete muscle-balancing resistance workout schedule to follow for all four weeks of Phase I. But before we get to that, let's go over the exercises involved.

There are 24 muscle-balancing resistance exercises, divided evenly among three categories: legs, core, and upper body. Here we go.

LEG EXERCISES

There are 8 muscle-balancing resistance workouts for the legs. They differ in terms of specific muscles targeted and equipment required.

Romanian Deadlift

MUSCLES TARGETED: hamstrings

REQUIRED EQUIPMENT: dumbbells

Stand with your feet close together, knees bent very slightly, with a dumbbell next to each foot. Set your core. Bend forward from the waist and grab the dumbbells. Return to a standing position with your arms at your sides, keeping your knees locked in the same slightly bent position. You'll feel that your hamstrings do most of the work in this movement. Pause briefly in a standing position and then bend forward to do another repetition.

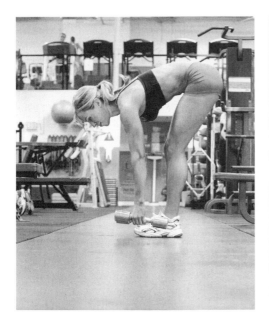 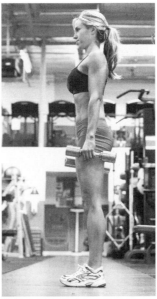

Wall Squat

MUSCLES TARGETED: quadriceps

EQUIPMENT REQUIRED: none

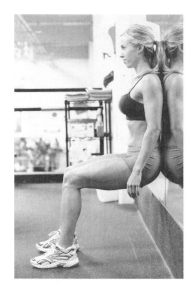

Set your core. Rest your back against a wall and squat down until your thighs are parallel to the floor. Hold this position until you feel a nice burn in the muscles on the front of your thighs. For a slightly greater challenge you can do this exercise with a stability ball positioned between your back and the wall.

Lying Hip Adduction

MUSCLES TARGETED: hips

EQUIPMENT REQUIRED: none

Lie on your left side with your torso propped up by both arms with your left leg fully extended and your right leg sharply bent and rotated so that your right foot is flat on the floor in front of your pelvic area. Set your core. Contract the muscles on the inner side of your left thigh and lift your left foot as high above the floor as possible. Pause briefly at the top of the movement and then return to the starting position. After completing a full set, reverse your position and work the right leg.

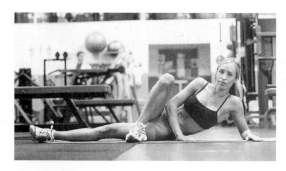
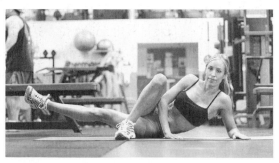

Standing Single-Leg Squat

MUSCLES TARGETED: quadriceps, buttocks

EQUIPMENT REQUIRED: exercise bench (dumbbells optional)

Set your core. Stand facing away from an exercise bench on your right foot only and rest the top of your left foot on the bench behind you. Slowly bend your right knee and squat down toward the floor, going as far down as you can without discomfort. Keep your back posture neutral and your weight on the heel of your right foot. Now push back upward to the starting position. After completing a full set, work the left leg. To make this exercise more challenging, do it while holding dumbbells at your sides.

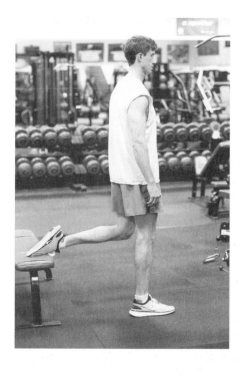
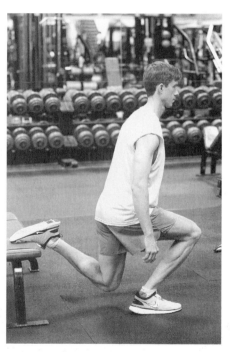

Heel Raise

MUSCLES TARGETED: calves

EQUIPMENT REQUIRED: exercise bench (dumbbells optional)

Stand facing an exercise bench with your hands on your hips. Set your core. Place your left foot on top of the bench. Contract your right calf and raise the heel off the floor as far as possible, pause briefly, and then lower it again. Complete a full set and then work your left calf. If you can do more than 15 repetitions without too much trouble, do this exercise while holding dumbbells at your sides.

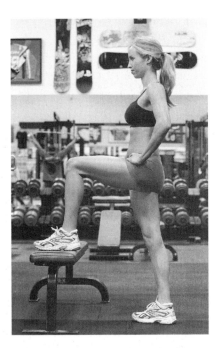 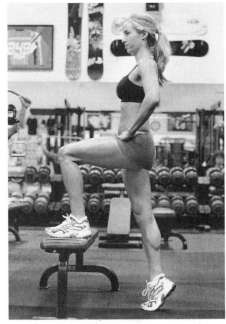

Side Step-Up

MUSCLES TARGETED: quadriceps, hips

EQUIPMENT REQUIRED: exercise bench, dumbbell

Stand with your right side facing an exercise bench while holding a dumbbell in your left hand with your left arm relaxed at your side. Set your core. Place your right foot on the bench and then straighten your right leg completely so you're now standing on the bench with your left leg unsupported. Be sure not to push off the floor with your left ankle—make your right leg do all the work of lifting your body to the height of the bench. Now step back down. After completing a full set, reverse your position and repeat with your left leg doing the work.

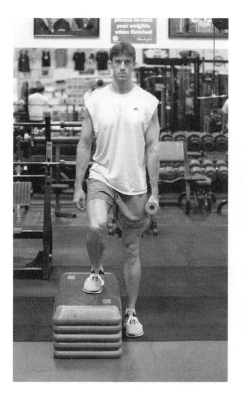
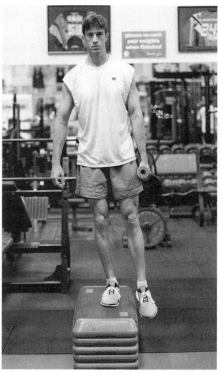

Heel Dip

MUSCLES TARGETED: calves

EQUIPMENT REQUIRED: none (regular staircase step)

Set your core. Balance on your left foot on a stair step with the ball of the foot resting on the edge of the stair so that the heel is unsupported. Rest your fingertips against a wall or some other support for balance. Lower your heel toward the floor until you feel a stretch in your calf muscles, then raise your heel back to a neutral position. Do 8 to 16 repetitions and then work your right calf.

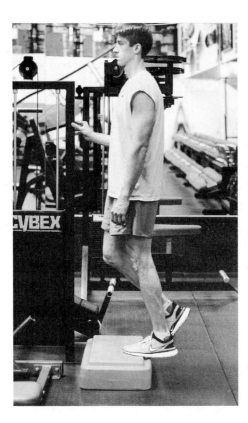 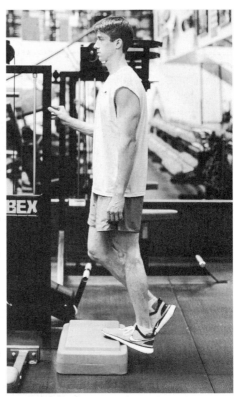

Double-Leg Buck

MUSCLES TARGETED: hamstrings

EQUIPMENT REQUIRED: exercise bench (or chair)

Lie faceup on the floor with your heels on an elevated platform such as an exercise bench and your legs bent at 90 degrees. (If you don't have an exercise bench you can use a chair.) Set your core. Contract your hamstrings, drive your heels into the platform, and lift your butt and torso upward until your body forms a straight line from knees to neck. Pause briefly and then return to the starting position. To make this exercise more challenging, perform a single leg buck, with only one foot in contact with the platform and the other foot elevated above it.

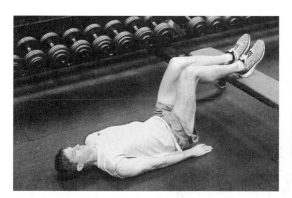
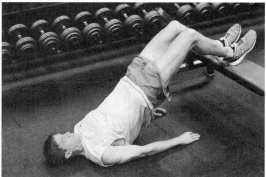

CORE EXERCISES

There are 8 total muscle balancing resistance workouts for the core. They differ in terms of specific muscles targeted and equipment required.

Dumbbell Row

MUSCLES TARGETED: mid-back

EQUIPMENT REQUIRED: dumbbell

Stand with your left foot one big step ahead of your right. Set your core. Bend both knees moderately and lean forward about 30 degrees from the waist. Brace your left hand on your lower left thigh. Grasp a dumbbell in your right hand and begin with your right arm fully extended toward the floor. Pull the dumbbell toward a spot just outside your lower rib cage, keeping your elbow in. Now slowly lower the dumbbell. After completing a full set, reverse your stance and switch arms.

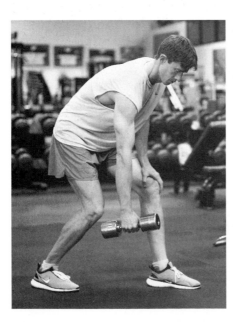 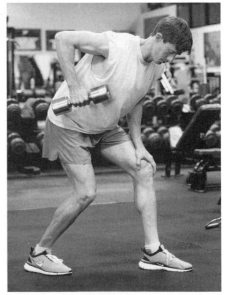

Cable Pull-down

MUSCLES TARGETED: mid-back

EQUIPMENT REQUIRED: cable resistance

Kneel on the floor facing a door gym or cable pulley station, about 2½ feet away from it. Set your core. Raise your right arm straight overhead and grasp a handle that's connected to the high attachment point. Keeping your arm completely straight, pull the handle toward the floor as far as possible. Pause briefly and return to the starting position. After completing a full set, switch arms.

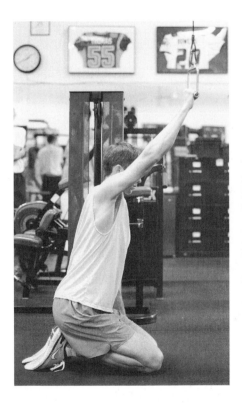 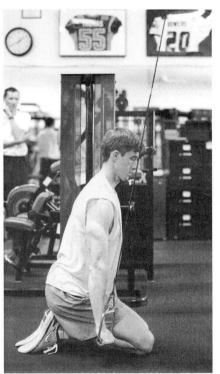

Stick Crunch

MUSCLES TARGETED: outer abs

EQUIPMENT REQUIRED: none (broomstick)

Lie on your back, bend your knees, and draw them as close to your chest as possible. Set your core. Grasp any type of stick or rod (such as a broom handle) with both hands positioned shoulder width apart. Begin with your arms extended straight toward your toes. Now squeeze your abdominal muscles and draw your chest and knees together until the stick passes beyond your toes. Pause for one second and relax. Do 15 to 30 repetitions.

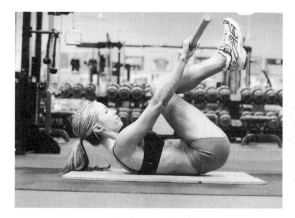 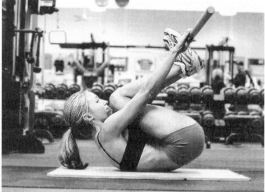

Oblique Crunch

MUSCLES TARGETED: outer abs, obliques

EQUIPMENT REQUIRED: none

Lie face up on the floor. Set your core. Raise your head and upper shoulders off the mat just slightly and lace the fingers of both hands together behind your head for support, keeping your elbows wide. Bend your knees 90 degrees and raise your feet an inch or two above the floor, as well. Contract your stomach muscles and at the same time twist your torso to the right, so your left elbow moves toward your left knee. Pause at the height of the movement and then return to the starting position without allowing your working muscles to relax completely. Alternate between leftward and rightward twists.

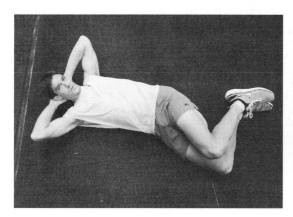 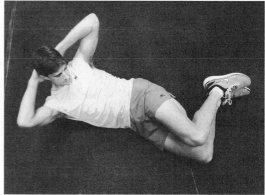

Superman

MUSCLES TARGETED: lower back

EQUIPMENT REQUIRED: none

Lie facedown with your arms outstretched Superman style. Set your core. Inhale and contract the muscles of your lower back and buttocks so that your head, arms, upper torso and legs come off the floor simultaneously, making a gentle U shape of your body. Hold this position for a 2-count and relax. Repeat 10 to 15 times.

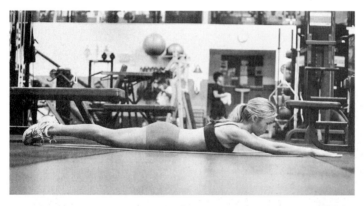

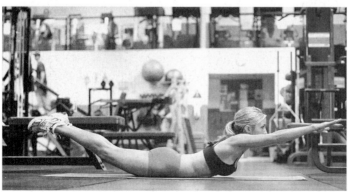

Good Morning

MUSCLES TARGETED: lower back

EQUIPMENT REQUIRED: dumbbells

Stand tall with your feet placed slightly farther than shoulder width apart and your arms extended straight upward. Set your core. Bend forward at the waist (avoid rounding your back) and reach the dumbbells toward your toes, going as far as you can without bending at the knees. Try to keep your arms more or less in line with your torso all the way down. Now return slowly to the upright position, standing tall with arms overhead. Again, maintain a neutral spine. *Do not perform this exercise if you have a history of lower-back injury or if you have any reason to believe you might be prone to lower-back pain.*

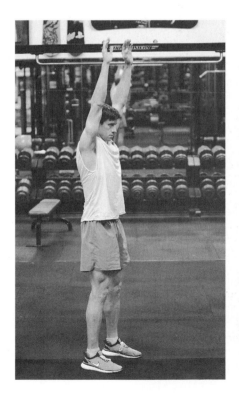 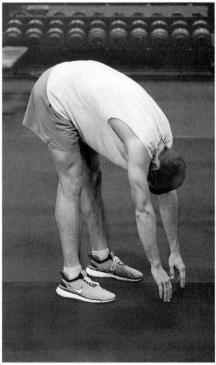

wrong back—don't round upper body parallel to floor

Side Plank

MUSCLES TARGETED: deep abs, obliques

EQUIPMENT REQUIRED: none

Lie on your right side with your ankles together and your torso propped up by your forearm. Set your core. Lift your hips upward until your body forms a diagonal plank from ankles to neck. Hold this position for 20 seconds, concentrating on not allowing your hips to sag toward the floor. (You might want to watch yourself in a mirror.) Reverse your position and repeat. Progress by increasing how long you hold the bridge position.

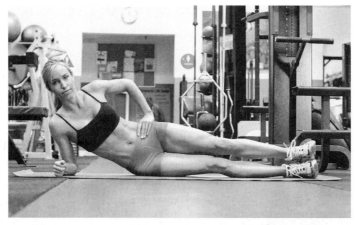

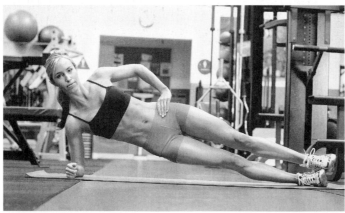

Stability Ball Crunch

MUSCLES TARGETED: outer abs

EQUIPMENT REQUIRED: stability ball

Lie face up with a stability ball supporting your hips, lower back and mid-back. Place your feet on the floor in a wide stance and bend your legs to 90 degrees. Set your core. Cross your arms over your chest and rest each hand on the opposite shoulder. Curl forward by trying to shorten the distance between the bottom of your rib cage and your hip bones. Bring your upper torso up to about 45 degrees from horizontal and then return to the starting position. Do not try to generate momentum by yanking your neck forward to start the crunch. Also avoid letting your abs relax at the bottom of the movement. To make this exercise more difficult, place your hands behind your head.

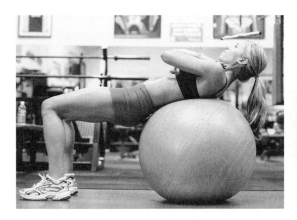 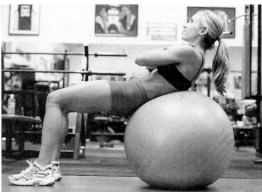

UPPER BODY EXERCISES

There are 8 total muscle-balancing resistance exercises for the upper body. They differ in terms of specific muscles targeted and equipment required.

Dumbbell Flye

MUSCLES TARGETED: chest

EQUIPMENT REQUIRED: exercise bench and dumbbells

Lie faceup on an exercise bench with your back flat. Bend your knees and place your feet flat on the end of the bench. Begin with your arms extended straight toward the ceiling, a dumbbell in each hand, and your palms facing each other. Set your core. Inhale as you slowly swing your arms out to the sides and toward the floor, bending your elbows slightly to protect them and stopping when you feel a comfortable stretch in your chest. Now, while exhaling, reverse direction and press the dumbbells back together overhead.

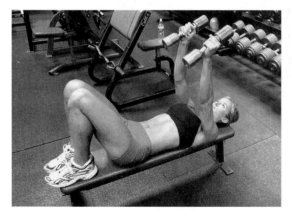 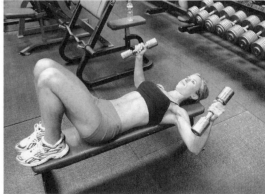

Shoulder Press

MUSCLES TARGETED: rear shoulders

EQUIPMENT REQUIRED: dumbbells

Stand comfortably with a dumbbell in each hand. Begin with your arms bent at the elbows at 90 degrees, your upper arms parallel to the floor, and your palms facing forward. Set your core. Now press the dumbbells toward the ceiling, extending your elbows fully. Pause briefly and return to the starting position.

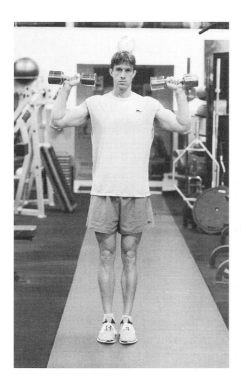
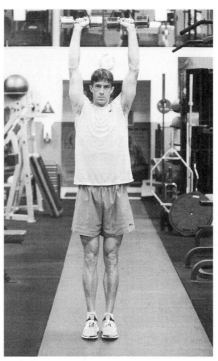

Shoulder Shrug

MUSCLES TARGETED: upper back

EQUIPMENT REQUIRED: dumbbells

Stand comfortably with your arms at your sides and a heavy dumbbell in each hand. Set your core. Lift your shoulders straight up toward your ears by contracting the muscles of your upper back. Keep your elbows in. Pause for 1 second at the top of the movement and then return to the starting position.

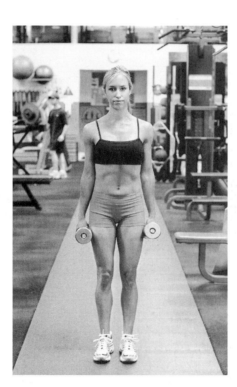 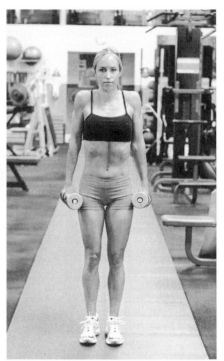

Push-up

MUSCLES TARGETED: chest, triceps, upper back

EQUIPMENT REQUIRED: none

Assume a normal push-up position with your hands placed shoulder width apart, your legs and back straight, feet together, and elbows locked. Look forward instead of at the ground. Set your core. Keeping your back straight, lower your chest until it almost touches the floor, then push smoothly back upward to the starting position. Maintain a moderate, controlled tempo. If you cannot complete 8 push-ups with good form, do a modified push-up with your knees touching the floor instead of your toes.

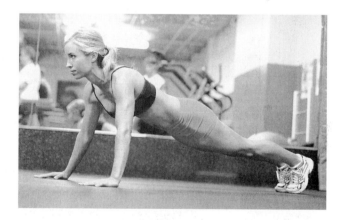

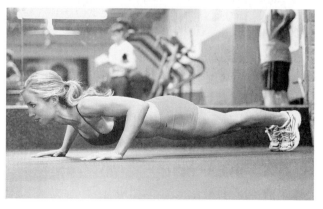

Side Shoulder Raise

MUSCLES TARGETED: mid-shoulders

EQUIPMENT REQUIRED: dumbbells

Stand normally with your arms at your sides and a dumbbell in each hand, palms in. Set your core. Lift your arms straight out to the sides, going slightly beyond the point where they are parallel to the floor. Slowly return to the starting position.

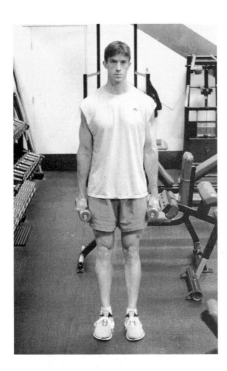
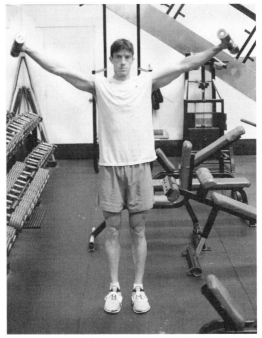

Cable Side Shoulder Raise

MUSCLES TARGETED: mid-shoulders

EQUIPMENT REQUIRED: cable resistance

Stand with your left side facing a door gym or cable pulley station. Connect a handle to the low attachment point and grasp it in your right hand. Begin with your arm extended straight downward in front of your right thigh with your palm facing the door or cable pulley station. Set your core. Contract your shoulder muscles and lift your arm straight outward, going just past the point where the arm is parallel to the floor. Pause briefly and return to the starting position. After completing a full set, work the left shoulder.

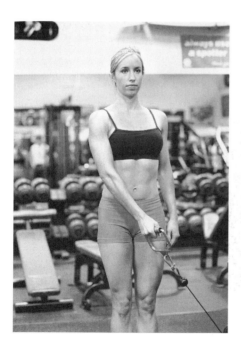
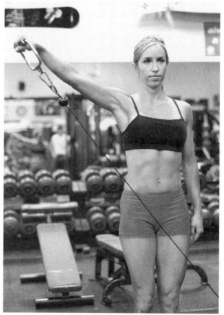

Cable Front Shoulder Raise

MUSCLES TARGETED: front shoulders

Equipment required: cable resistance

Stand facing away from a door gym or cable pulley station. Connect a handle to the low attachment point and grasp it in your right hand with your right arm relaxed at your side, palm facing the door or cable pulley station. Set your core. Contract the muscles on the front of your shoulder and lift the handle forward and upward, going just past the point where your arm is parallel to the floor. Pause briefly and return to the starting position. After completing a full set, work the left shoulder.

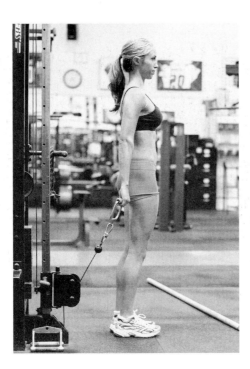
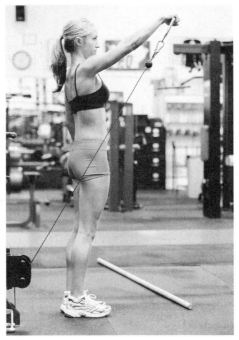

Upright Cable Row

MUSCLES TARGETED: upper back

EQUIPMENT REQUIRED: cable resistance

Stand facing a door gym or cable pulley station with two handles connected to low attachment points. Grasp each handle with an overhand grip and begin with your arms extended straight toward the floor and your inner wrists touching the front of your thighs. Set your core. Now bend your elbows, draw them wide apart, and pull the handles straight upward toward your chin. Pause briefly at the top of the movement and return to the starting position.

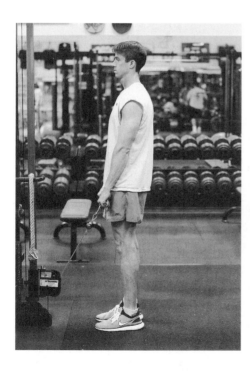
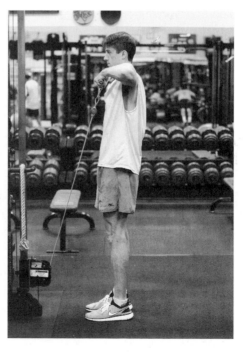

MUSCLE-BALANCING WORKOUTS

You are free to put together your own muscle-balancing resistance workouts using exercises of your choice. Remember to start with the warm-up described earlier in the chapter. Do not rest between exercises. Instead, without rushing, complete one exercise and immediately set up for the next exercise and move straight into it. Also do not hurry your performance of individual exercises. By simply not resting between exercises you are doing enough to keep your breathing and calorie burning rates high. Rushing the exercises will only lessen the muscle-developing benefit of the workout and put you at risk of injury.

There are two considerations that will factor into the exercises you select. First you will have to work around exercises that require equipment you don't have access to. In addition, try to avoid choosing multiple exercises that challenge the same muscles within each area of the body. For example, don't include both the heel raise and the heel dip, both of which challenge the calves. Your circuits need to target all of the major muscle groups of the body. Some overlap is acceptable, as long as no muscle group is left unchallenged by the workout. The following summary of all 24 muscle-balancing resistance exercises will help you put together balanced circuits.

If you prefer not to trouble yourself with creating your own muscle-balancing resistance workouts, then simply select ready-made workouts from among the following ones I've put together for you. There are four workouts in total: two beginner workouts (nine exercises each) involving different equipment and two advanced workouts (12 exercises each) involving different equipment.

SUMMARY OF MUSCLE-BALANCING RESISTANCE EXERCISES

Exercise	Type	Equipment	Muscles Targeted
Romanian Deadlift	Legs	Dumbbells	Hamstrings
Wall Squat	Legs	None	Hamstrings
Lying Hip Adduction	Legs	None	Hips
Standing Single Leg Squat	Legs	Exercise bench (dumbbells optional)	Quadriceps, buttocks
Heel Raise	Legs	Exercise bench (dumbbells optional)	Calves
Side Step-up	Legs	Exercise bench (dumbells optional)	Quadriceps, hips
Heel Dip	Legs	None (regular stair step)	Calves
Double-leg Buck	Legs	Exercise bench (or chair)	Hamstrings
Dumbbell Row	Core	Dumbbell	Mid-back
Cable Pull-down	Core	Cable Resistance	Mid-back
Stick Crunch	Core	None (broomstick)	Outer abs
Oblique Crunch	Core	None	Outer abs, obliques
Superman	Core	None	Lower back
Good Morning	Core	Dumbbells	Lower back
Side Plank	Core	None	Deep abs, obliques
Stability Ball Crunch	Core	Stability Ball	Outer abs
Dumbbell Flye	Upper Body	Exercise bench, dumbbells	Chest
Shoulder Press	Upper Body	Dumbbells	Rear shoulders
Shoulder Shrug	Upper Body	Dumbbells	Upper back
Push-up	Upper Body	None	Chest, triceps, upper back
Side Shoulder Raise	Upper Body	Dumbbells	Mid-shoulders
Cable Side Shoulder Raise	Upper Body	Cable Resistance	Mid-shoulders
Cable Front Shoulder Raise	Upper Body	Cable Resistance	Front shoulders
Upright Cable Row	Upper Body	Cable Resistance	Upper back

PHASE I

91

BEGINNER MUSCLE-BALANCING WORKOUT #1 (9 EXERCISES)

Equipment: stability ball and cable resistance

Leg Exercise #1	Wall Squat (page 68)
Core Exercise #1	Cable Pull-down (page 75)
Upper Body Exercise #1	Push-up (page 85)
Leg Exercise #2	Lying Hip Adduction (page 68)
Core Exercise #2	Stick Crunch (page 76)
Upper Body Exercise #2	Cable Side Shoulder Raise (page 87)
Leg Exercise #3	Heel Dip (page 72)
Core Exercise #3	Superman (page 78)
Upper Body Exercise #3	Cable Front Shoulder Raise (page 88)

BEGINNER MUSCLE-BALANCING WORKOUT #2 (9 EXERCISES)

Equipment: exercise bench and dumbbells

Leg Exercise #1	Romanian Deadlift (page 67)
Core Exercise #1	Dumbbell Row (page 74)
Upper Body Exercise #1	Dumbbell Flye (page 82)
Leg Exercise #2	Standing Single Leg Squat (page 69)
Core Exercise #2	Stick Crunch (page 76)
Upper Body Exercise #2	Shoulder Press (page 83)
Leg Exercise #3	Heel Raise (page 70)
Core Exercise #3	Good Morning (page 79)
Upper Body Exercise #3	Shoulder Shrug (page 84)

ADVANCED MUSCLE-BALANCING WORKOUT #1 (12 EXERCISES)

Equipment: stability ball and cable resistance

Leg Exercise #1	Wall Squat (page 68)
Core Exercise #1	Cable Pull-down (page 75)
Upper Body Exercise #1	Push-up (page 85)
Leg Exercise #2	Lying Hip Adduction (page 68)
Core Exercise #2	Stick Crunch (page 76)
Upper Body Exercise #2	Cable Side Shoulder Raise (page 88)
Leg Exercise #3	Heel Dip (page 72)
Core Exercise #3	Superman (page 78)
Upper Body Exercise #3	Cable Front Shoulder Raise (page 88)
Leg Exercise #4	Double-Leg Buck (with chair) (page 73)
Core Exercise #4	Stability Ball Crunch (page 81)
Upper Body Exercise #4	Upright Cable Row (page 89)

ADVANCED MUSCLE-BALANCING WORKOUT #2 (12 EXERCISES)

Equipment: exercise bench and dumbbells

Leg Exercise #1	Romanian Deadlift (page 67)
Core Exercise #1	Dumbbell Row (page 74)
Upper Body Exercise #1	Dumbbell Flye (page 82)
Leg Exercise #2	Standing Single Leg Squat (page 69)
Core Exercise #2	Stick Crunch (page 76)
Upper Body Exercise #2	Shoulder Press (page 83)
Leg Exercise #3	Heel Raise (page 70)
Core Exercise #3	Good Morning (page 79)
Upper Body Exercise #3	Shoulder Shrug (page. 84)
Leg Exercise #4	Side Step-up (page 71)
Core Exercise #4	Side Plank (page 80)
Upper Body Exercise #4	Side Shoulder Raise (page 86)

DETAILED PHASE I RESISTANCE WORKOUT SCHEDULES

The following charts present detailed resistance workout schedules for all of Phase I for both the beginner and the advanced levels. I have only prescribed workout templates. You may create actual workouts by filling them in with specific exercises selected from the pool of 24 muscle-balancing resistance exercises. Alternatively, you may use an appropriate ready-made workout.

BEGINNER SCHEDULE

Wk #	Monday	Wednesday	Friday
1	Resistance (Muscle Balancing) Summary 1 circuit 9 exercises 12 minutes Workout: Warm-up 1X* Leg exercise #1 Core exercise #1 Upper body exercise #1 Leg exercise #2 Core exercise #2 Upper body exercise #2 Leg exercise #3 Core exercise #3 Upper body exercise #3	Resistance (Muscle Balancing) Summary 1 circuit 9 exercises 12 minutes Workout: Warm-up 1X* Leg exercise #1 Core exercise #1 Upper body exercise #1 Leg exercise #2 Core exercise #2 Upper body exercise #2 Leg exercise #3 Core exercise #3 Upper body exercise #3	Resistance (Muscle Balancing) Summary 1 circuit 9 exercises 12 minutes Workout: Warm-up 1X* Leg exercise #1 Core exercise #1 Upper body exercise #1 Leg exercise #2 Core exercise #2 Upper body exercise #2 Leg exercise #3 Core exercise #3 Upper body exercise #3
2	Resistance (Muscle Balancing) Summary 1 circuit 9 exercises 12 minutes Workout: Warm-up 1X* Leg exercise #1 Core exercise #1	Resistance (Muscle Balancing) Summary 1 circuit 9 exercises 12 minutes Workout: Warm-up 1X* Leg exercise #1 Core exercise #1	Resistance (Muscle Balancing) Summary 1 circuit 9 exercises 12 minutes Workout: Warm-up 1X* Leg exercise #1 Core exercise #1

* 1X=1 complete circuit (i.e., do one set of each exercise).

Wk #	Monday	Wednesday	Friday
	Upper body exercise #1 Leg exercise #2 Core exercise #2 Upper body exercise #2 Leg exercise #3 Core exercise #3 Upper body exercise #3	Upper body exercise #1 Leg exercise #2 Core exercise #2 Upper body exercise #2 Leg exercise #3 Core exercise #3 Upper body exercise #3	Upper body exercise #1 Leg exercise #2 Core exercise #2 Upper body exercise #2 Leg exercise #3 Core exercise #3 Upper body exercise #3
3	Resistance (Muscle Balancing) Summary 2 circuits 9 exercises 21 minutes Workout: Warm-up 2X** Leg exercise #1 Core exercise #1 Upper body exercise #1 Leg exercise #2 Core exercise #2 Upper body exercise #2 Leg exercise #3 Core exercise #3 Upper body exercise #3	Resistance (Muscle Balancing) Summary 2 circuits 9 exercises 21 minutes Workout: Warm-up 2X* Leg exercise #1 Core exercise #1 Upper body exercise #1 Leg exercise #2 Core exercise #2 Upper body exercise #2 Leg exercise #3 Core exercise #3 Upper body exercise #3	Resistance (Muscle Balancing) Summary 2 circuits 9 exercises 21 minutes Workout: Warm-up 2X* Leg exercise #1 Core exercise #1 Upper body exercise #1 Leg exercise #2 Core exercise #2 Upper body exercise #2 Leg exercise #3 Core exercise #3 Upper body exercise #3
4	Resistance (Muscle Balancing) Summary 1 circuit 9 exercises 12 minutes Workout: Warm-up 1X* Leg exercise #1 Core exercise #1 Upper body exercise #1 Leg exercise #2 Core exercise #2 Upper body exercise #2 Leg exercise #3 Core exercise #3 Upper body exercise #3	Resistance (Muscle Balancing) Summary 1 circuit 9 exercises 12 minutes Workout: Warm-up 1X* Leg exercise #1 Core exercise #1 Upper body exercise #1 Leg exercise #2 Core exercise #2 Upper body exercise #2 Leg exercise #3 Core exercise #3 Upper body exercise #3	Resistance (Muscle Balancing) Summary 1 circuit 9 exercises 12 minutes Workout: Warm-up 1X* Leg exercise #1 Core exercise #1 Upper body exercise #1 Leg exercise #2 Core exercise #2 Upper body exercise #2 Leg exercise #3 Core exercise #3 Upper body exercise #3

** 2X=2 complete circuits (i.e., do the full sequence of exercises twice).

ADVANCED SCHEDULE

Wk #	Monday	Wednesday	Friday
1	Resistance (Muscle Balancing) Summary 1 circuit 12 exercises 15 minutes Workout: Warm-up 1X Leg exercise #1 Core exercise #1 Upper body exercise #1 Leg exercise #2 Core exercise #2 Upper body exercise #2 Leg exercise #3 Core exercise #3 Upper body exercise #3 Leg exercise #4 Core exercise #4 Upper body exercise #4	Resistance (Muscle Balancing) Summary 1 circuit 12 exercises 15 minutes Workout: Warm-up 1X Leg exercise #1 Core exercise #1 Upper body exercise #1 Leg exercise #2 Core exercise #2 Upper body exercise #2 Leg exercise #3 Core exercise #3 Upper body exercise #3 Leg exercise #4 Core exercise #4 Upper body exercise #4	Resistance (Muscle Balancing) Summary 1 circuit 12 exercises 15 minutes Workout: Warm-up 1X Leg exercise #1 Core exercise #1 Upper body exercise #1 Leg exercise #2 Core exercise #2 Upper body exercise #2 Leg exercise #3 Core exercise #3 Upper body exercise #3 Leg exercise #4 Core exercise #4 Upper body exercise #4
2	Resistance (Muscle Balancing) Summary 1 circuit 12 exercises 15 minutes Workout: Warm-up 1X Leg exercise #1 Core exercise #1 Upper body exercise #1 Leg exercise #2 Core exercise #2 Upper body exercise #2 Leg exercise #3 Core exercise #3 Upper body exercise #3 Leg exercise #4 Core exercise #4 Upper body exercise #4	Resistance (Muscle Balancing) Summary 1 circuit 12 exercises 15 minutes Workout: Warm-up 1X Leg exercise #1 Core exercise #1 Upper body exercise #1 Leg exercise #2 Core exercise #2 Upper body exercise #2 Leg exercise #3 Core exercise #3 Upper body exercise #3 Leg exercise #4 Core exercise #4 Upper body exercise #4	Resistance (Muscle Balancing) Summary 1 circuit 12 exercises 15 minutes Workout: Warm-up 1X Leg exercise #1 Core exercise #1 Upper body exercise #1 Leg exercise #2 Core exercise #2 Upper body exercise #2 Leg exercise #3 Core exercise #3 Upper body exercise #3 Leg exercise #4 Core exercise #4 Upper body exercise #4

* 1X=1 complete circuit (i.e., do one set of each exercise).

Wk #	Monday	Wednesday	Friday
3	Resistance (Muscle Balancing)	Resistance (Muscle Balancing)	Resistance (Muscle Balancing)
	Summary 2 circuits 12 exercises 27 minutes	Summary 2 circuits 12 exercises 27 minutes	Summary 2 circuits 12 exercises 27 minutes
	Workout: Warm-up 2X Leg exercise #1 Core exercise #1 Upper body exercise #1 Leg exercise #2 Core exercise #2 Upper body exercise #2 Leg exercise #3 Core exercise #3 Upper body exercise #3 Leg exercise #4 Core exercise #4 Upper body exercise #4	Workout: Warm-up 2X Leg exercise #1 Core exercise #1 Upper body exercise #1 Leg exercise #2 Core exercise #2 Upper body exercise #2 Leg exercise #3 Core exercise #3 Upper body exercise #3 Leg exercise #4 Core exercise #4 Upper body exercise #4	Workout: Warm-up 2X Leg exercise #1 Core exercise #1 Upper body exercise #1 Leg exercise #2 Core exercise #2 Upper body exercise #2 Leg exercise #3 Core exercise #3 Upper body exercise #3 Leg exercise #4 Core exercise #4 Upper body exercise #4
4	Resistance (Muscle Balancing)	Resistance (Muscle Balancing)	Resistance (Muscle Balancing)
	Summary 1 circuit 12 exercises 15 minutes	Summary 1 circuit 12 exercises 15 minutes	Summary 1 circuit 12 exercises 15 minutes
	Workout: Warm-up 1X Leg exercise #1 Core exercise #1 Upper body exercise #1 Leg exercise #2 Core exercise #2 Upper body exercise #2 Leg exercise #3 Core exercise #3 Upper body exercise #3 Leg exercise #4 Core exercise #4 Upper body exercise #4	Workout: Warm-up 1X Leg exercise #1 Core exercise #1 Upper body exercise #1 Leg exercise #2 Core exercise #2 Upper body exercise #2 Leg exercise #3 Core exercise #3 Upper body exercise #3 Leg exercise #4 Core exercise #4 Upper body exercise #4	Workout: Warm-up 1X Leg exercise #1 Core exercise #1 Upper body exercise #1 Leg exercise #2 Core exercise #2 Upper body exercise #2 Leg exercise #3 Core exercise #3 Upper body exercise #3 Leg exercise #4 Core exercise #4 Upper body exercise #4

** 2X=2 complete circuits (i.e., do the full sequence of exercises twice).

CHAPTER 7

Cardio Exercise:

Short Intervals

People are always asking me about the best form of cardio exercise. By "best" they mean the most effective for fat burning and the most time efficient. My response is always the same: "You're asking the wrong question!" There are many forms of cardio exercise that are more or less equally effective. The important question is, Which one do you enjoy doing the most? Which one will you be able to stick with? After all, no form of cardio exercise is effective if you stop doing it!

The Lean Look cardio workouts can be applied to many popular forms of cardio exercise, and I encourage you to adapt the workouts I prescribe to your preferred form. In fact, you can even practice more than one form of cardio exercise. Many of my clients do, and they find that variation helps them stay motivated and avoid overuse injuries. In this chapter I will discuss the advantages and disadvantages of six specific types of cardio training—bicycling, elliptical training and stair climbing, inline skating, running, swimming, and walking—and provide tips on how to get started in each. If you already have a favorite, don't let me steer you away from it. But if you're open to various possibilities, this information will help you make the best choice for your program.

Later in the chapter I will describe the three specific types of interval workouts that you will perform in the cardio component of Phase I and provide workout schedules for both the beginner and advanced levels.

THERE'S MORE THAN ONE WAY TO TRIM THE FAT

Bicycling (indoors or outdoors), elliptical training and stair climbing, inline skating, running, swimming, and walking are all excellent cardio activities. The one that's best for you might not be the best choice for someone else. Here's everything you need to know to get started in the right direction.

BICYCLING

Bicycling has many advantages: It burns calories at a high rate; it's easy and convenient; it carries a low injury risk; and it tones up the leg muscles. In addition, bicycling lends itself especially well to the sorts of high-intensity intervals that you'll do in Phase I. Just pedal faster and/or increase your gear ratio or resistance level when you start the interval and do the opposite at the end of the interval. You can do this riding outdoors or on a stationary bike at home or at the gym.

In order to do any outdoor riding, you need a bike, of course. There are many different kinds of bikes; which is best for you depends primarily on your intended use for it. If you want a bike that's light enough and has enough gears to get you up and over hills, but you also want some comfort and you don't intend to use it for racing, your best choice would be a comfort bike or a hybrid. If you plan to do some rough off-road riding, you'll need a cross-country mountain bike. (Comfort bikes and hybrids can handle light off-road use.) If you intend to ride on pavement exclusively and you want something fast, use a road bike or a time trial bike. Comfort and hybrid bikes are generally the least expensive; you can get a new bike from a reputable manufacturer for about $350. Mountain bikes are a little more expensive, starting in the $600 range. Road bikes are more expensive still ($1,000 at entry level).

Take care when shopping for a bike. The best first move you can make is to choose a good shop. The best bike shops have honest, knowledgeable salespeople who make a genuine effort to match you up with the best bike for your needs. Such shops are in the minority, so be sure to do a little research before you decide where to buy. Comfort and fit are crucial considerations in choosing the right bike, and the fit factor is tricky enough that you could very easily purchase an ill-fitting or poorly adjusted bike if your salesperson is not well trained or just doesn't care.

A helmet is mandatory equipment for outdoor cycling. Sports sunglasses are virtually a must-have, as well. If you ride a high-performance road bike with a lightweight seat, you will almost certainly want to wear padded bike shorts, which will make the riding experience infinitely more comfortable. And if you're at all serious about your riding it's best that you use cycling shoes that clip onto the pedals and allow you to generate force more evenly throughout the pedal stroke. I strongly recommend that on every ride you carry the items needed to replace or repair a punctured inner tube, and that you learn how to use them. (Most any bike shop mechanic will gladly show you.) One last equipment item that is very handy is a bike computer that is affixed to the handlebar and records distance traveled, tells you how fast you're going, and so forth. You can get a basic one for less than $50.

Important skills that you will need to learn in order to ride safely and/or proficiently include positioning (there are several hand positions you can use on a road bike), pedaling mechanics, gear selection, climbing, descending, braking, and cornering. You will develop a feel for each of these skills simply through accumulating experience on the bike. However, you can accelerate the learning process by learning them from a more experienced cyclist, coach, cycling magazine, book, or Web site.

If you plan to ride indoors you have a few options. Most health clubs offer a selection of high-quality stationary bikes you can use. You can also purchase a stationary bike for home use from an exercise equipment retailer. A well-built model from a reputable manufacturer such as Schwinn or Life Fitness will cost you $500 or more. A cheaper alternative is to buy a "bike trainer" on which you can mount your regular bike for stationary indoor use. The two best types of bike trainers are magnetic trainers and fluid trainers; they are available at most performance-oriented bike shops (i.e., bike shops where competitive cyclists and triathletes shop) starting at roughly $100.

ELLIPTICAL TRAINING AND STAIR CLIMBING

The four most popular types of cardio exercise machines are elliptical trainers, stationary bikes, stair climbers, and treadmills. I've already mentioned stationary bikes, and I'll discuss treadmills in the running section later in the chapter.

The elliptical trainer was invented in the 1990s by the fitness equipment maker Precor, which sought to design a machine that closely simulated the action of running without impact. As a result, elliptical trainers combine the fat-burning power of running and the low injury risk of nonimpact activities such as bicycling. Now manufactured by a number of companies, elliptical trainers have become standard equipment in health clubs.

Elliptical trainer models vary widely in their design, quality, and features. Most health clubs provide high-quality machines that work well for all users. If you wish to purchase an elliptical trainer for home use, your first consideration is budget. The least expensive machines cost about $400. Health club–quality machines usually cost upward of $3,000. The more expensive machines tend to have a more fluid, natural stride motion and far fewer breakdowns than the cheaper ones. The pricier machines are motor driven, whereas the most affordable ones are not. Motor-driven machines are almost always smoother and also offer variable resistance (and variable incline, too, in some models), which is essential if you want to vary your effort level by pace and resistance level. But these machines must be plugged into a wall socket before you can operate them.

Once you've settled on a price range, visit stores and try various machines within that price range. Pick the machine that feels most fluid and comfortable as you operate it. Other considerations include display and programming features, quietness, size and storage, and warranty and service. Try to choose a machine with an easy-to-read display that allows you to manually adjust resistance (and incline, if applicable) without much fuss. Nearly all motor-driven elliptical trainers come with preprogrammed workouts, but since you are going to follow my Lean Look workouts, you might be more interested in a machine that allows you to add workouts, such as the speed intervals, power intervals, and 1-minute intervals you'll do in Phase I.

Some machines are quieter than others, and it's always nice to get a quiet unit if you can. In addition, there is quite a bit of variation in how much floor space various machines take up, and you'll want to be sure the machine you buy will actually fit in the space you have in mind for it. A few models fold for storage between workouts. Finally, ask your salesperson what sort of warranty is offered on the machine and how it will be serviced if anything should go wrong with it, and be sure you're comfortable with his or her answers before you pull out your credit card.

Some elliptical trainers have moving handles that allow you to work your upper body muscles against resistance, while others have a fixed handle that is used for balance. Neither type is inherently better than the other, and both types are equally easy to use. However, there is one common error that many people make on elliptical trainers with a fixed handle: They lean heavily on it while working out. You'll get a better workout if you stand fully upright while using your elliptical trainer and put just enough pressure on the handle with your fingers to maintain your balance. Better still, practice swinging your arms in opposition to your leg movements as you would when running.

Stair-climbers have lost a lot of popularity to elliptical trainers, but a stair-climbing machine offers a workout that's very similar to that of an elliptical trainer, and it is no less effective. As with elliptical trainers, high-quality stair-climbers are available at many fitness clubs. Expect to pay at least $2,000 to purchase a stair-climber of equal quality for home use. Nonmotorized stair-climbers using hydraulic resistance are available for as little as $600, but they lack the fluid feel of the more costly motorized units. The other big quality difference among stair-climbers has to do with the "stairs" themselves. Most models feature levered foot pedals that move up and down to simulate a stair-climbing motion. A few others feature a rotating belt with actual steps that you have to lift your feet onto. One disadvantage of rotating belts is that the size of the stairs cannot be adjusted for individuals of different heights, whereas with levered pedals you can take steps of any size. Another disadvantage of rotating belts is that they don't offer variable resistance, so you can adjust the intensity of exercise only by stepping faster or slower.

As on elliptical trainers, many users of stair-climbers make the mistake of leaning heavily on the machine's handrails, which lessens your weight bearing while exercising and makes the workout easier and less effective than it should be. Another common error on stair-climbers is taking abnormally large steps; this should be avoided because it places undue stress on the knee joints.

INLINE SKATING

The great thing about inline skating is that it's fun. It has many of the same virtues as running, yet it's *faster,* and there's something ineffably satisfying about the feeling of gliding. The main disadvantage of skating is that it's no fun at all unless you're on a very smooth surface and you know how to skate, so you're much more limited in terms of where you can go on skates than you are if you're on foot. Inclement weather is also more likely to foil skating than running. However, you can get around this problem by purchasing a slide board such as the Powerslide that allows you to "skate" (slide from side to side on a slick board) in place (wearing socks or fabric booties) indoors. Slide boards typically cost $125 to $200.

Outdoor skating requires skates, of course. Many varieties are sold; the kind you want is the kind called *fitness skates.* Yes, there are racing skates, featuring five wheels instead of four and a longer wheelbase, but these are best avoided by beginners and even intermediate skaters. Expect to pay between $110 and $170 for a high-quality pair of new fitness skates. The best place to buy them is at a specialty store from a salesperson who skates rather than at one of those sporting goods megastores. Tell the salesperson where and how you intend to use them, ask for his or her recommendations, and try on at least three models. The fit should be quite snug but not constricting.

Wheel types and sizes vary even more than do the skates themselves. Larger and harder wheels tend to be faster while smaller and softer wheels tend to offer more control. Wheels wear more quickly on the outside edge, so you'll need to rotate your wheels when they begin to look worn on that side (it's very easy) and replace them once they're worn on both sides. Buy a helmet at the same time you buy your skates and wear it for every skating work-out. Hand and wrist pads are recommended for all skaters as well, and beginners will also want to wear knee and elbow pads.

If you are a beginner, before you start doing actual workouts on inline skates you need to devote a couple of sessions to practicing three basic skills: striding, stopping, and falling. The stride comes quickly. Find a flat, smooth surface and begin by getting your stance right. Bend your knees a little and shift most of your weight onto your heels. If you can't lift your toes to the top of the boot, your center of gravity is too far forward. Form a V with your skates and begin walking forward, maintaining the V. Use your arms for balance.

Once you get comfortable walking on skates, start trying to glide a bit. Begin with both skates in full contact with the ground in the V shape and push off with the left skate to make the right skate glide diagonally forward. Touch down with the left skate and then push off with the right to glide on the left. Keep trying to glide farther and farther, seeing how far you can go on one skate. Once you're able to glide with steady balance, try skating with one hand grasping the opposite wrist behind your back, as doing so is more energy efficient than anything else you might do with your arms.

There are three common braking systems on inline skates. The most common is a rubber pad and plastic arm attached to the heel of your skate. (On most good models the brake arm may be attached to either skate; put it on your dominant side.) To use the brake, position your feet side by side, slide the braking skate forward, and then dip your heel toward the ground until the rubber pad makes contact and begins to drag. This asymmetrical drag and the deceleration it causes will challenge your balance at first, so start slowly. Some beginners find it helpful to practice balancing on one skate before they practice braking. There are fancier ways to brake, such as V stops and hockey stops, but you should master this basic stop before you try any others.

Falling is all but inevitable for beginners. Unless you practice correct falling technique, you will fall incorrectly at first and experience more pain than is necessary. Skaters usually fall backward. This is the worst way to fall, because you'll almost certainly hit rear end first and really jar your tailbone. And from there you could very well fall back and whack your head. When you begin to fall backward, twist around to one side as you go and try to absorb the impact on the knee and elbow pads on that side. Splitting the impact fifty-fifty in this manner will greatly reduce your chance of injury. Find a grassy spot and practice turning a backward fall into a side fall. If you ever fall forward, don't throw your arms out and take the impact on your hands, as most skaters instinctively do. Instead throw your knees down and land first on your kneepads, *then* throw your arms out and *slide* forward on your hands and knees, keeping your torso off the pavement.

Another potential disadvantage of inline skating is that it may be harder to adapt the high-intensity intervals of Phase I to this activity than to some of the other cardio activities discussed in this chapter. Doing short intervals near or at maximum intensity on inline skates will require that you skate at a very high rate of speed or skate up a hill (which will necessitate your skating back down the hill between intervals). I don't think either of these options is very attractive to the inexperienced inline skater, so you might want to try another type of cardio exercise for Phase I.

RUNNING

Running remains one of the most popular forms of exercise, and for good reason: It is extremely effective and you can do it just about anywhere, anytime, with minimal equipment. Running provides a great cardiovascular workout in a short amount of time, and in terms of fitness bang for the buck it's hard to beat. You'll also find it quite easy to adapt the Phase I workouts to running. Just speed up and/or start running uphill to start an interval and do the opposite at the end of the interval.

Although running is notoriously unpleasant for beginners, once you've got the hang of it, running can be a primal pleasure, as attested to by the famous "runner's high" that many people experience. Running is a very natural movement. Look at how much running children do. There's an urge to run in all of us, and satisfying that urge feels good.

The main disadvantage of running is that it has a high injury rate, due in large part to the high-impact nature of the activity. Overuse injuries such as bone strains, stress fractures, and knee pain are all too common, especially among beginners. To avoid them you need to build your running mileage very gradually so that your bones, muscles, and joints have the opportunity to adapt to the stress. In fact, I don't recommend that you use running as your cardio workout of choice in the Lean Look program unless you have done some running recently. If you have not been running at least somewhat regularly in recent weeks and you want to run in the Lean Look program, give yourself at least three or four weeks to adapt to running before you start the program. Start by doing walks with short, slow jogging intervals lasting 1 minute apiece. Gradually increase the duration of the jogging intervals until you're able to run for 20 minutes without experiencing abnormal pain during or between workouts.

It's also important to choose your shoes carefully. Have a knowledgeable running shoe expert analyze your stride in order to match you with the right shoe. Use your running shoes for running only and replace them every 400–600 miles. Varying the types of surface you run on may help prevent injuries, too.

A treadmill is one "surface" choice you're free to choose if you have access to such a machine and you don't want to run outside in foul weather or for any other reason. Virtually every health club has high-quality treadmills. You can buy a well-built treadmill for home use for $1,500 to $3,000. There are big differences in quality and features among the various models, so I recommend that you discuss the options with a knowledgeable salesperson and try several models before you buy.

SWIMMING

A swimming workout burns as many calories as a bike ride and enhances cardiorespiratory health and fitness as well as running does. As a full-body exercise, it conditions every major muscle group from your shoulders to your ankles, and because it is performed against the resistance of water, swimming improves strength as well as endurance. But unlike other forms of exercise, swimming is not only nonimpact but also non–weight bearing, so it's easy on the bones and joints.

Once you've decided to start swimming, the first thing you need to do is find a good place to swim. You can locate lap pools in your area by flipping through the yellow pages, asking friends and acquaintances who swim, or visiting the United States Masters Swimming Web site (www.usms.org). Some facilities allow you to pay by the visit (usually $5 or so), while others require a membership. Before committing to a membership, try the facility to see whether it's clean, pleasant, and accessible enough for your needs. It's also important to find a pool that is not too crowded at the times you like to work out.

As for equipment, the essentials are a swimsuit and goggles, which you can find at any sporting goods store, and a swim cap, if your hair is long enough to obstruct your vision when wet. Other handy items are a swim duffel bag with compartments for wet and dry gear, antifogging drops for your goggles, and pool sandals.

There are four common swim strokes: freestyle, breaststroke, backstroke, and butterfly. Most swimmers spend most of their time practicing freestyle, as it covers the greatest distance in the least time. Proper freestyle technique does not come automatically to anyone, but anyone can learn it. There are five basic elements of good freestyle form.

• **High float.** It's important to float high in the water, as doing so minimizes drag. Beginners tend to allow their hips and legs to sink. To avoid this error, concentrate on pushing your chest toward the bottom of the pool. Your hips and legs will automatically rise.

• **Body rotation.** By rotating your entire body from side to side with each stroke, you swim more narrowly and can slice through the water with less drag. As you extend your leading arm ahead of you, rotate your body about 60 degrees toward the opposite side (as though you're reaching to pluck an item off a high shelf). But be sure to keep your neck and head neutral.

• **High elbow pull.** Once you've reached full extension with your leading arm, rotate your shoulder and elbow so that your hand and forearm form a single "paddle" that pulls back toward your feet. A proper high elbow pull is often described as feeling like "reaching over a barrel."

• **Long strokes.** Long strokes mean more distance traveled per stroke. Be sure to pull all the way back until your arm is fully extended toward your foot. Your hand should exit the water next to your upper thigh.

• **Efficient kick.** Kicking too hard will create more drag than it does propulsion, so concentrate on making a tight, small, "flicking" kick that uses minimal energy. The proper motion is similar to that of kicking a ball, but you're moving your foot only 6 inches in either direction. Kick four times, twice with each leg, for each stroke you make with your arms.

If you're not an experienced swimmer, understand that it will take some time to develop an efficient freestyle stroke. Be patient and keep working at it. If possible, ask an experienced swimmer or swim coach to watch you swim and point out errors you're making so you can correct them. This is a never-ending process. Even Olympic swimmers are constantly fine-tuning their technique. The good news is that the less efficient your swimming stroke is, the more calories you burn in getting from one end of the pool to the other!

A crucial difference between swimming and every other form of cardio exercise discussed in this chapter is that you can't monitor time while swimming, which makes it a little trickier to perform precisely timed swimming intervals. The secret is to learn how many strokes you take or how many pool lengths you cover in a given period of time at a given effort level. For example, for your 1-minute interval workouts (described later in the chapter), which feature 1-minute hard intervals and 1-minute active recoveries, figure out how many strokes you complete in 1 minute while swimming at an appropriately hard level of effort. Then you will be able to perform this workout properly by counting in your head instead of referring to a stopwatch.

WALKING

Walking is an excellent alternative to running for those who are unable to run without pain and for those who are not yet fit enough for running. It is probably not the best choice for you if you are moderately fit already, because you will find it hard to crank the intensity level high enough—especially for power intervals—without breaking into a run. Nevertheless, you can make walking more challenging than you might think it can be by doing your intervals on a very steep hill.

One of the nice things about walking is that it does not require any fancy or expensive equipment. However, certain clothes and shoes are better suited to fitness walking than others, and it is important that you use gear that is designed for this use.

Unfortunately, most shoes sold as "walking shoes" are too stiff and heavy for more than a few miles of easy strolling (on carpet, in a mall, etc.). If you try to wear these clunky white cowhide "nursing shoes" during a long training walk you'll end up with hot, sweaty, blistered feet. A lightweight, flexible running shoe with a relatively low heel is a much better choice for most walkers.

Look for the following characteristics when shopping for walking shoes:

• **Flexibility.** Your shoes must be flexible enough to allow your feet to "roll" from heel to toe when you walk or you'll wind up with sore shins.

• **Low heel.** The bigger the heel on the shoe, the more your feet will slap the ground when you walk. With a low heel your feet will roll very easily along the ground.

• **Wide toe box.** Make sure there's plenty of "wiggle room" for your toes to spread out as you walk. Cramped toes will become blistered toes.

• **Custom fit.** The most important consideration is the way the shoes fit *your* feet. When shopping for shoes, wear the same socks as well as any shoe inserts or orthotics you will wear walking. Also be aware that your feet will swell during the day, so try on shoes late in the day—preferably after a work-out—when your feet are at their largest. Don't be afraid to walk around the store to make sure the shoes fit in action.

Once you've found your perfect shoe, consider buying a second pair. Alternating shoes from day to day will extend their life and ensure that you'll always have a dry pair. You may even want to try another model or brand for your second pair since different shoes will change your walking mechanics enough to work slightly different muscles.

Entire books have been written about walking technique, but the best advice can be summed up in two words: walk naturally. Stand up straight, don't swing your arms wildly or take very long strides and you'll do just fine.

PHASE I CARDIO WORKOUTS

As I first mentioned back in chapter 3, all of the cardio workouts in the Lean Look program are interval workouts, meaning their format consists of short, high-intensity bursts of activity separated by periods of lower-intensity "active recovery." Interval workouts are a staple in the training programs of all competitive endurance athletes. Swimmers do interval workouts in the pool, cyclists do them on the road, and runners do them on the track, but the formats are essentially the same in each sport. The reason is simple: Interval workouts are an incredibly effective way to boost performance in any endurance discipline. So it was inevitable that they would be discovered, and once discovered maintained, in every endurance sport. But you don't have to be a competitive endurance athlete to benefit from interval workouts. They are also the best form of cardio exercise if your goal is to get lean.

It's a fundamental rule of human performance that the faster you go, the sooner you become fatigued. And the slower you go, the longer you can continue before fatigue sets in. In short, speed and duration are somewhat incompatible, which is too bad, because each is beneficial for fat burning and fitness building. Going faster—or raising the intensity of exercise—accelerates calorie burning and enhances the cardiovascular and performance benefits of cardio exercise. But exercising for a longer time increases the total benefit of exercise at any intensity. Is it possible to get the benefits of speed and duration from a single cardio workout?

You bet. Interval workouts find a compromise between going faster and exercising for a longer time by inserting low-intensity "active recovery" periods between short segments of high-intensity activity (or intervals). Breaking your high-intensity cardio exercise into short segments enables you to do more total exercise at high intensity within a single workout than you could do if you simply maintained a high intensity without interruption until you became exhausted. Inserting low-intensity active recoveries between intervals enables you to recover enough to take on another hard interval while still keeping your metabolism elevated (as compared to resting completely between intervals). In this way, intervals combine the advantages of slow, steady cardio workouts and short, high-intensity workouts. A complete interval cycle is comprised of one hard (high-intensity) interval, followed by one active recovery interval.

For example, you might do a workout consisting of 6 high-intensity intervals lasting 1 minute apiece, alternating with six 1-minute active recovery intervals. The intensity of the high-intensity 1-minute intervals is determined using the plus-one rule: You do each 1-minute interval at the highest level of effort you could sustain through one more high-intensity interval than you will actually do. Since this particular example workout calls for you to do 6 high-intensity intervals, you would do each high-intensity interval at the highest effort level you could sustain through 7 intervals. Now, if you actually worked at this intensity level without any active recoveries, you would probably be completely exhausted after just 4 minutes and done for the day. But by doing 1-minute intervals at this high intensity you can delay exhaustion until you've completed 6 high-intensity intervals, or a total of 6 minutes, at this intensity. Consequently, this workout will be more beneficial than a 4-minute non-interval workout at the same high intensity. Plus, the interval workout will be extended by 6 active recoveries of 1 minute apiece. Although these active recoveries are done at a very gentle pace, they still add 6 minutes of elevated metabolism to your workout.

Many of my clients come to me with little or no prior experience in doing cardio intervals. Any cardio training they've done in the past has been of the slow-and-steady variety. These folks are often amazed by the results they get from interval workouts, and by how time efficient these workouts are. A typical example is Ernie, who came to me as a thirty-nine-year-old father, husband, and regional supervisor for a home improvement store. Ernie wanted help losing weight (he started at 275 pounds) and overcoming a bad knee. The only way he knew to shed body fat was to do long, slow cardio workouts, such as the miles of running he had done in his military days. But his knee couldn't handle it, especially at his size.

Because Ernie lived in the mountains and traveled frequently, I helped him select exercise equipment to purchase for his home: a stationary bike, elliptical trainer, free weights, medicine balls, a Swiss ball, bands, and a treadmill. I also suggested that he dust off his hiking boots and road bike. I showed him that by doing short, high-intensity bursts of activity and stringing them together with low-intensity recovery periods, his workouts could be fun and pain-free. As time went on and he began to drop weight and get in better shape, I gradually increased the duration of Ernie's cardio sessions. Once he saw that he could burn calories and shed fat without having to spend 90 minutes on the treadmill, he was completely sold on this way of training, and he's still at it.

There are various interval workout formats. The main variables are the duration and the intensity of each interval. Obviously, shorter intervals can be done at higher intensities, while lower-intensity intervals can be sustained longer. When beginning a new exercise program, it's best to do interval workouts featuring very short intervals performed at near-maximum intensity. Studies have shown that these workouts are better tolerated by men and women of a lower fitness level than are slightly longer intervals done at a slightly lower intensity. Such workouts also produce the fastest fitness gains for such individuals. Even if your current level of cardiovascular fitness is pretty good, you can still reap huge benefits from focusing on short intervals for a few weeks.

You will do three types of short interval workouts in Phase I of the Lean Look program: speed intervals on Tuesdays, 1-minute intervals on Thursdays, and power intervals on Saturdays. (Remember, you'll do resistance workouts on Mondays, Wednesdays, and Fridays.)

Speed intervals are 30-second high-intensity intervals followed by 1-minute active recoveries. *Power intervals* are 20-second high-intensity intervals followed by 2-minute active recoveries. And *1-minute intervals* are 1-minute moderately high-intensity intervals followed by 1-minute active recoveries. Begin each cardio workout with a 5-minute warm-up performed at a moderate effort level in your chosen cardio activity and finish with a 5-minute cooldown at the same intensity. Perform your active recoveries at the same level of effort as your warm-up and cooldown. Resist any temptation you may feel to shorten your warm-up or do it at a high intensity. Beginning each cardio workout with a thorough, comfortable warm-up is very important because it warms, lubricates, and oxygenates the muscles, preparing them to perform better and with less strain in the high-intensity intervals to follow.

In the following pages are specific guidelines for each of the three cardio interval workouts you will do in Phase I of the Lean Look program.

SPEED INTERVALS

This workout will take 16 to 22 minutes to complete, depending on the number of intervals you do. (For instance, the speed intervals workout in Week 1 of the beginner schedule consists of 4 speed intervals totaling 16 minutes, while the speed intervals workout in Week 3 of the advanced schedule consists of 8 speed intervals totaling 22 minutes.)

To do a speed intervals workout, first warm up with 5 minutes of moderate-intensity movement in your chosen activity. Next increase your effort to a very high level for 30 seconds. Use the plus-one rule to determine the appropriate level of effort for the high-intensity interval: That is, aim for the highest possible level of effort you could sustain through one more interval than the workout requires.

Depending on your choice of activity, you can increase the level of effort not only by increasing your pace but also by increasing the level of resistance. For example, if you're running or walking (either outdoors or on a treadmill), you might time each 30-second high-intensity interval to coincide with the start of a hill climb (gravitational resistance). If you're on a bike, you might switch to a high gear ratio (outdoors) or higher resistance level (stationary bike). If you're using an elliptical trainer or stair climber, you might increase the climbing gradient and/or resistance level at the beginning of each high-intensity interval. By using increased resistance in combination with increased tempo to achieve a high level of effort, you reduce the likelihood of injury as compared to using increased tempo alone to produce a maximal effort, which could result in a strained muscle or tendon.

After completing a 30-second interval, slow back down to your warm-up pace for 1 minute. You've just completed one speed interval cycle. After completing the prescribed number of intervals, cool down at your warm-up effort level for 5 minutes. Do not perform a 1-minute active recovery following your last speed interval, but instead go straight to the cooldown. Thus a speed intervals workout featuring four interval cycles looks like this ("hard" equals "high-intensity"):

5-minute easy warm-up

30 seconds hard

1-minute active recovery

30 seconds hard

1-minute active recovery

30 seconds hard

1-minute active recovery

30 seconds hard

5-minute easy cooldown

Total time: 15:00

POWER INTERVALS

This interval workout takes 18 to 26 minutes to complete, depending on the number of intervals prescribed in the specific workout you're doing.

Power intervals are very similar to speed intervals, except that (a) the intensity level is even higher—very close to your absolute maximum; (b) the high-intensity intervals are therefore necessarily slightly shorter (20 seconds); (c) you will achieve maximal effort primarily by working against higher resistance (as I'll explain presently) and only secondarily by picking up your cadence; and (d) the active recovery periods are longer (2 minutes) to give you plenty of opportunity to get ready for the next power interval. Here's how to do this workout.

First, warm up with 5 minutes of moderate-intensity movement in your chosen activity. Next increase your effort level to near maximum for 20 seconds. Use the plus-one rule to guide your effort. Increase your effort level by increasing your tempo and resistance, but put the emphasis on increasing the resistance. If you're walking or running, do your power intervals on a steep hill. If you're bicycling, do them on a steep hill or put your bike in its highest gear. If you're swimming, wear hand paddles. If you're using an elliptical trainer, increase the gradient and/or resistance. If you're using a stair climber with adjustable resistance, crank up the resistance. Power is a combination of speed and strength, so increasing the resistance in your power intervals is an important way to emphasize the strength component. Try to stay relaxed and maintain good form in your activity. Don't flail or push yourself to the point where you risk straining a muscle or tendon.

After completing the 20-second power interval, reduce your effort level back down to your warm-up level for 2 minutes. After completing the prescribed number of 20-second power intervals, cool down for 5 minutes. Do not perform a 2-minute active recovery following your last power interval, but instead go straight to the cooldown. Thus a power intervals workout featuring 4 intervals looks like this:

5-minute easy warm-up

20 seconds hard

2-minute active recovery

20 seconds hard

2-minute active recovery

20 seconds hard

2-minute active recovery

20 seconds hard

5-minute easy cooldown

Total time: 17:20 (17 minutes rounded)

1-MINUTE INTERVALS

This interval workout takes 17 to 29 minutes to complete, depending on the number of intervals you do. The 1-minute intervals workout in Week 1 of the beginner schedule consists of four speed intervals for a workout totaling 17 minutes. The longest 1-minute intervals workout actually occurs in Phase II of the advanced schedule; it consists of ten 1-minute intervals and the workout takes 29 minutes.

To do a 1-minute intervals workout, first warm up with 5 minutes of moderate-intensity movement in your chosen activity. Next increase your effort level by increasing your pace and/or resistance for 1 minute. Use the plus-one rule to guide your level of effort. After completing the 1-minute interval, slow back down to your warm-up effort level for 1 minute. Once you've completed the prescribed number of 1-minute intervals, cool down for 5 minutes. Do not perform a 1-minute active recovery following your last 1-minute interval, but instead go straight to the cooldown. Thus, a 1-minute intervals workout featuring 4 intervals looks like this:

5-minute easy warm-up

1 minute hard

1-minute active recovery

1 minute hard

1-minute active recovery

1 minute hard

1-minute active recovery

1 minute hard

5-minute easy cooldown

Total time: 17 minutes

If you have not done short intervals such as these before, it might take you one or two workouts to find just the right pace, resistance level, and effort level at which to perform the intervals. In terms of effort level, you'll know you've got it right if you complete the last prescribed interval at the same pace at which you started the first one and are feeling as if you could complete one (and only one) more high-intensity interval at the same pace if you had to. Before long you will have a good feel for what constitutes a proper level of effort for the high-intensity intervals in the speed, power, and 1-minute interval workouts and how much to increase your tempo and resistance level when doing high-intensity intervals in each type of interval workout.

Finding the right combination of tempo and resistance is an individual matter and also depends on your specific choice of activity. If your chosen activity is one you've been doing for a while, finding the right pace will come fairly quickly. If it's a new activity, it may take a little longer. In any case, approach the first workout of each type as a trial run and try to err on the side of caution.

The following charts provide detailed Phase I cardio workout schedules for the beginner level and the advanced level. The high-intensity intervals of all three types—speed intervals, power intervals, and 1-minute intervals—are designated by the word "hard," but remember that the precise level of effort should be slightly different for each type of workout.

PHASE 1 CARDIO EXERCISE—BEGINNER SCHEDULE

Wk #	Tuesday	Thursday	Saturday
1	Speed Intervals 5-minute easy warm-up 4 X (30 seconds hard/ 1 minute easy) 5-minute easy cooldown Total time: 15 minutes	1-Minute Intervals 5-minute easy warm-up 4 X (1 minute hard/ 1 minute easy) 5-minute easy cooldown Total time: 17 minutes	Power Intervals 5-minute easy warm-up 4 X (20 seconds hard/ 2 minutes easy) 5-minute easy cooldown Total time: 18 minutes
2	Speed Intervals 5-minute easy warm-up 5 X (30 seconds hard/ 1 minute easy) 5-minute easy cooldown Total time: 17 minutes	1-Minute Intervals 5-minute easy warm-up 5 X (1 minute hard/ 1 minute easy) 5-minute easy cooldown Total time: 19 minutes	Power Intervals 5-minute easy warm-up 5 X (20 seconds hard/ 2 minutes easy) 5-minute easy cooldown Total time: 21 minutes
3	Speed Intervals 5-minute easy warm-up 6 X (30 seconds hard/ 1 minute easy) 5-minute easy cooldown Total time: 18 minutes	1-Minute Intervals 5-minute easy warm-up 6 X (1 minute hard/ 1 minute easy) 5-minute easy cooldown Total time: 21 minutes	Power Intervals 5-minute easy warm-up 6 X (20 seconds hard/ 2 minutes easy) 5-minute easy cooldown Total time: 23 minutes
4	Speed Intervals 5-minute easy warm-up 4 X (30 seconds hard/ 1 minute easy) 5-minute easy cooldown Total time: 15 minutes	1-Minute Intervals 5-minute easy warm-up 4 X (1 minute hard/ 1 minute easy) 5-minute easy cooldown Total time: 17 minutes	Power Intervals 5-minute easy warm-up 4 X (20 seconds hard/ 2 minutes easy) 5-minute easy cooldown Total time: 18 minutes

PHASE 1 CARDIO EXERCISE—ADVANCED SCHEDULE

Wk #	Tuesday	Thursday	Saturday
1	Speed Intervals 5-minute easy warm-up 6 X (30 seconds hard/ 1 minute easy) 5-minute easy cooldown Total time: 19 minutes	1-Minute Intervals 5-minute easy warm-up 6 X (1 minute hard/ 1 minute easy) 5-minute easy cooldown Total time: 21 minutes	Power Intervals 5-minute easy warm-up 6 X (20 seconds hard/ 2 minutes easy) 5-minute easy cooldown Total time: 23 minutes
2	Speed Intervals 5-minute easy warm-up 7 X (30 seconds hard/ 1 minute easy) 5-minute easy cooldown Total time: 20 minutes	1-Minute Intervals 5-minute easy warm-up 7 X (1 minute hard/ 1 minute easy) 5-minute easy cooldown Total time: 23 minutes	Power Intervals 5-minute easy warm-up 7 X (20 seconds hard/ 2 minutes easy) 5-minute easy cooldown Total time: 26 minutes
3	Speed Intervals 5-minute easy warm-up 8 X (30 seconds hard/ 1 minute easy) 5-minute easy cooldown Total time: 21 minutes	1-Minute Intervals 5-minute easy warm-up 8 X (1 minute hard/ 1 minute easy) 5-minute easy cooldown Total time: 25 minutes	Power Intervals 5-minute easy warm-up 8 X (20 seconds hard/ 2 minutes easy) 5-minute easy cooldown Total time: 28 minutes
4	Speed Intervals 5-minute easy warm-up 6 X (30 seconds hard/ 1 minute easy) 5-minute easy cooldown Total time: 19 minutes	1-Minute Intervals 5-minute easy warm-up 6 X (1 minute hard/ 1 minute easy) 5-minute easy cooldown Total time: 21 minutes	Power Intervals 5-minute easy warm-up 6 X (20 seconds hard/ 2 minutes easy) 5-minute easy cooldown Total time: 23 minutes

PHASE II

CHAPTER 8

Introduction to Phase II

I n Phase II of the Lean Look program you will begin to practice eight nutrient timing habits while continuing to practice the key food substitutions you began using in Phase I. You will also continue to perform three resistance workouts and three cardio workouts, but the nature of these workouts will change.

The focus of your resistance workouts will shift from muscle balancing to strength building. On the cardio side, you will incorporate two new interval workouts (2-minute and 3-minute intervals) while phasing out the speed and power interval workouts you did in Phase I. Finally, don't forget to measure your body fat percentage once a week throughout Phase II, as you did in the first four weeks of the program.

NUTRITION: NUTRIENT TIMING

Nutrition scientists have recently discovered that *when* we eat and drink is almost as important as *what* we eat and drink. Specifically, we need to time our energy (i.e., calorie) consumption to coincide with our energy needs. Nutrient timing is a set of habits that are designed to achieve this objective. There are eight specific nutrient timing habits that you will begin practicing in Phase II of the Lean Look program.

Most of these changes are fairly subtle, but they can add up to make a big difference in accelerating your progress. As I mentioned before, if you are strongly motivated to do so, you may begin to practice nutrient timing in Phase I alongside your key substitutions. Otherwise it's best to wait until Week 5 to begin practicing nutrient timing, to avoid feeling overwhelmed by changing too many of your nutrition habits too suddenly.

RESISTANCE EXERCISE: STRENGTH BUILDING

The resistance workouts you did in Phase I were designed to create a solid foundation for future muscle development. In Phase II you will begin doing resistance workouts that are designed to build on this foundation by increasing your strength. The strength gains you achieve in doing these workouts will be accompanied by muscle growth, which will in turn increase your metabolic rate and promote fat burning.

Throughout Phase II you will do two strength-building resistance workouts per week (on Mondays and Fridays) that are made up of the new exercises presented in chapter 10. On Wednesdays you will continue to do a muscle-balancing resistance workout to help you maintain the foundation you developed in Phase I.

CARDIO EXERCISE: INTERMEDIATE INTERVALS

The three cardio workouts you did in Phase I featured short or relatively short intervals. This approach to cardio training is appropriate for the first few weeks of a new exercise program, because it produces fast results in a way that is not too challenging for those who are not yet very fit. Slightly longer intervals of 2 or 3 minutes, performed at a slightly lower but still high level of effort, are more challenging and therefore best suited to those who have had a few weeks to build a foundation of cardio fitness with shorter intervals. But because they are more challenging, 2- and 3-minute intervals are also very effective in taking one's cardio fitness and leanness to the next level.

In Phase II you will do cardio workouts featuring 2-minute intervals on Tuesdays and cardio workouts featuring 3-minute intervals on Saturdays; I'll explain this in chapter 11. On Thursdays you will continue to do cardio workouts featuring 1-minute intervals, as you did in Phase I.

As you can see, we're building on Phase I; all the work you do in each phase will continue to pay off throughout the program.

WORKOUT SCHEDULES

On the following pages are general resistance and cardio workout schedules for Phase II of the Lean Look program. Chapters 10 and 11 provide more detailed information about how to do your Phase II resistance workouts and cardio workouts. After you have finished reading through all of the text on Phase II, refer back to the tables provided here, which show you how your resistance workouts and cardio workouts fit together week by week.

BEGINNER SCHEDULE

The following chart lists the general Phase II resistance and cardio workout schedule for the beginner exercise level. Use this workout schedule if you started with the beginner schedule in Phase I, or if you started with the advanced schedule in Phase I but are finding the workouts too challenging or are having trouble recovering fully between workouts.

Wk #	Monday	Tuesday	Wednesday	Thursday	Friday	Saturday
5	Resistance (Strength Building)	Cardio (2-Minute Intervals)	Resistance (Muscle Balancing)	Cardio (1-Minute Intervals)	Resistance (Strength Building)	Cardio (3-Minute Intervals)
	2 circuits 9 exercises	4 intervals	2 circuits 9 exercises	6 intervals	2 circuits 9 exercises	3 intervals
	18 minutes	24 minutes	18 minutes	21 minutes	18 minutes	25 minutes
6	Resistance (Strength Building)	Cardio (2-Minute Intervals)	Resistance (Muscle Balancing)	Cardio (1-Minute Intervals)	Resistance (Strength Building)	Cardio (3-Minute Intervals)
	3 circuits 9 exercises	5 intervals	3 circuits 9 exercises	7 intervals	3 circuits 9 exercises	3 intervals
	27 minutes	28 minutes	27 minutes	23 minutes	27 minutes	25 minutes
7	Resistance (Strength Building)	Cardio (2-Minute Intervals)	Resistance (Muscle Balancing)	Cardio (1-Minute Intervals)	Resistance (Strength Building)	Cardio (3-Minute Intervals)
	3 circuits 9 exercises	5 intervals	3 circuits 9 exercises	8 intervals	3 circuits 9 exercises	4 intervals
	27 minutes	28 minutes	27 minutes	25 minutes	27 minutes	31 minutes
8	Resistance (Strength Building)	Cardio (2-Minute Intervals)	Resistance (Muscle Balancing)	Cardio (1-Minute Intervals)	Resistance (Strength Building)	Cardio (3-Minute Intervals)
	2 circuits 9 exercises	4 intervals	2 circuits 9 exercises	6 intervals	2 circuits 9 exercises	3 intervals
	18 minutes	24 minutes	18 minutes	21 minutes	18 minutes	25 minutes

ADVANCED SCHEDULE

The following chart lists the general Phase II resistance and cardio workout schedule for the advanced exercise level. Use this workout schedule if you started with the advanced schedule in Phase I and have not found the workouts in this schedule too challenging.

Wk #	Monday	Tuesday	Wednesday	Thursday	Friday	Saturday
5	Resistance (Strength Building)	Cardio (2-Minute Intervals)	Resistance (Muscle Balancing)	Cardio (1-Minute Intervals)	Resistance (Strength Building)	Cardio (3-Minute Intervals)
	2 circuits 12 exercises	5 intervals	2 circuits 12 exercises	8 intervals	2 circuits 12 exercises	4 intervals
	24 minutes	28 minutes	24 minutes	25 minutes	24 minutes	31 minutes
6	Resistance (Strength Building)	Cardio (2-Minute Intervals)	Resistance (Muscle Balancing)	Cardio (1-Minute Intervals)	Resistance (Strength Building)	Cardio (3-Minute Intervals)
	3 circuits 12 exercises	6 intervals	3 circuits 12 exercises	9 intervals	3 circuits 12 exercises	4 intervals
	36 minutes	32 minutes	36 minutes	27 minutes	36 minutes	31 minutes
7	Resistance (Strength Building)	Cardio (2-Minute Intervals)	Resistance (Muscle Balancing)	Cardio (1-Minute Intervals)	Resistance (Strength Building)	Cardio (3-Minute Intervals)
	3 circuits 12 exercises	6 intervals	3 circuits 12 exercises	10 intervals	3 circuits 12 exercises	5 intervals
	36 minutes	32 minutes	36 minutes	29 minutes	36 minutes	37 minutes
8	Resistance (Strength Building)	Cardio (2-Minute Intervals)	Resistance (Muscle Balancing)	Cardio (1-Minute Intervals)	Resistance (Strength Building)	Cardio (3-Minute Intervals)
	2 circuits 12 exercises	5 intervals	2 circuits 12 exercises	8 intervals	2 circuits 12 exercises	4 intervals
	24 minutes	28 minutes	24 minutes	25 minutes	24 minutes	31 minutes

CHAPTER 9

Nutrition: Nutrient Timing

Thousands of years ago, before the advent of agriculture, human beings had to work extremely hard for their food. They had to climb trees to gather nuts and berries and walk far afield in search of edible plants and roots, fleeing the occasional predator along the way. Hunting was even less efficient. Experts believe that men used more energy to complete a successful hunt than they got from the meat of the animals they killed.

The agricultural revolution (8000 BCE) is believed to have somewhat reduced the amount of energy people had to expend to bring food to the table. Primitive farming and animal husbandry were taxing work, but at least the food was nearby and, in good times, plentiful.

Beginning in the eighteenth century, the Industrial Revolution brought technological advances that made food cultivation and production much easier, and the trend continues in the twenty-first century. Nowadays only a small percentage of the population is directly involved in making food. The average person labors to obtain food only indirectly, perhaps by sitting in a chair and entering information into a computer forty hours a week to earn money that can be used to obtain food from supermarkets and restaurants. The amount of calories the average human being must burn to satisfy his or her hunger each day has decreased markedly since our hunter-gatherer days.

Before the modern age, a person's body typically needed food calories badly by the time the work required to acquire food was completed. Consequently very few people were fat. Today, by contrast, our energy needs and energy intake are far more loosely coupled, and as a result most of us are overweight. The moral of this history review is that the timing of energy intake matters. The energy we get from foods is put to the best use when our bodies actually need the energy at the time, and when we take in no more energy than we need to supply our immediate energy needs. If we take in food energy when we don't need it, or take in a lot when we need only a little (or when we don't take in energy when we do need it), problems result.

Our bodies use food calories very differently depending on how badly energy is needed (remember, a calorie is a unit of energy). Take the example of drinking a can of soda, which contains 140 calories of energy in the form of sugars. If you drink this can of soda with a meal after three hours of quietly watching television, a large portion of the sugars in the soda will be converted to triglycerides (fat) by the liver and stored in adipose tissue for later use, because you've burned very little energy recently and have taken in more than enough calories. However, if you consume the same can of soda 20 miles into a marathon, the sugars it contains will be hurried straight to the muscles of your legs and burned to fuel the last 6.2 miles to the finish line. Consequently those calories will be gone within minutes instead of stored in your belly for weeks, months, or years.

If you made your living as a hunter-gatherer or primitive farmer, your energy intake would be naturally well timed to meet short-term energy needs, except in times of scarcity. But we modern humans can't exactly improve our own nutrient timing patterns by going back to hunting, gathering, and primitive farming. What we can do instead is take advantage of the new science of nutrient timing to better balance our energy intake with our energy needs within the context of the modern lifestyle. Recent research has confirmed that *when* we eat and drink is almost as important as *what* we eat and drink with respect to the goal of optimizing body composition. By learning how to take advantage of the rules of nutrient timing, you can shed fat and gain muscle without any additional caloric restrictions once you've already made the key substitutions prescribed in Phase I. While this claim might sound too good to be true, there is a good deal of solid research to back it up. The effects of nutrient timing—whether your eating is well timed or poorly timed—are far greater than intuition tells us they should be. I have also seen ample proof of the effectiveness of proper nutrient timing in my hands-on work with clients.

Consider the example of one of my athlete clients, Stephanie, a twenty-four-year-old recreational triathlete. When I started working with Stephanie she was already fit and healthy, with solid dietary habits and a low, 18 percent body fat measurement. Her one complaint was that she was experiencing a lack of energy that was affecting her training. I looked into the timing of Stephanie's meals and quickly saw that she was not getting enough calories before and during her workouts to fuel performance, nor after workouts to speed her body's recovery from training. So we took roughly 300 total calories from her lunch and dinner and moved them to pre-workout and post-workout snacks.

After two weeks on this regimen, Stephanie came back to me and reported that she felt better during training and had even lost 2 pounds and 1 percent body fat. However, she was now feeling especially fatigued in the evening. After giving this new information some thought, I came to the conclusion that Stephanie's body had probably adapted to the poor nutrient timing of her past eating regimen by slowing her metabolism during and after workouts, which is probably why she felt lethargic in training. When we started fueling her workouts and recovery processes better, her body started burning all of the extra energy during her training, allowing her to perform better, and also burning it during the post-workout recovery period. But this left her in a state of energy deficit during the rest of the day, and that is why she lost weight and felt fatigued late in the day.

So we added 300 calories back to her lunch and dinner without removing them from the pre-workout and post-workout periods. And what happened? She felt great during her training and all day *and* she lost another 2 pounds in the next two weeks, as well as another 1 percent body fat. My final conclusion was that Stephanie had not been able to work to her full metabolic capacity due to poor nutrient timing and a slight energy deficit. Two years later she still feels great and remains at 16 percent body fat.

There are eight specific nutrient timing tips that I have found especially effective for both my athlete clients like Stephanie and my nonathlete clients who merely exercise to improve their bodies. They are as follows:

1. Rev up your metabolism by eating a good breakfast.
2. Keep your energy level consistent throughout the day with healthy snacks.
3. Bounce back faster after workouts with smart recovery nutrition.
4. Prevent overeating at meals by eating appetite-spoiling appetizers.
5. Fuel stronger workouts with the right pre-workout meals.
6. Prevent overeating at meals by eating slowly.
7. Build muscle overnight with a bedtime protein snack.
8. Fuel stronger workouts with sports drinks.

In the following sections I will explain why each of these nutrient timing measures is beneficial and I will provide detailed guidance on how to practice it. Your nutrition objective in Phase II of the Lean Look program is to incorporate into your daily eating habits any of these eight nutrient timing practices that you are not already taking advantage of. Naturally, once you begin practicing a new nutrient timing measure, you need to keep practicing it or you'll lose the benefits.

EIGHT WAYS TO MAKE NUTRIENT TIMING WORK FOR YOU

The following eight nutrient timing tips are presented in order of decreasing importance. This means that you should integrate them into your lifestyle in the order in which you encounter them here.

Nutrient Timing Tip #1: Rev Up Your Metabolism by Eating a Good Breakfast.

The rationale for nutrient timing is that our bodies make the best use of the energy we get from food when its intake coincides with peaks in our energy needs. In other words, we should eat more when our energy needs are greatest and less (or not at all) when our energy needs are least. By concentrating our energy intake during periods of high energy needs, we ensure that the majority of our food calories go toward satisfying immediate physiological requirements—such as supplying glucose to our brain so we can think, proteins to our muscles to regenerate tissues, and fats to cells throughout our body to support cell membranes—instead of going toward long-term storage in our visceral fat cells (i.e., the fat cells in our midsection, where fat accumulation is especially hazardous to long-term health).

It so happens that our energy needs tend to be greater in the morning than during the afternoon or evening. Therefore the first rule of nutrient timing is to start your day with a healthy breakfast providing at least 250 calories and eaten within an hour of waking up.

There are three reasons why our energy needs are greater in the morning. First, when we wake up in the morning we have not eaten for approximately twelve hours. Our central nervous system uses glucose throughout the night to keep running, so by the time the alarm goes off our liver is 50 percent depleted of glycogen (the storage form of glucose). Second, we tend to be more active during the first eight hours after waking than during the last eight hours before going to bed. And finally, our bodies actually burn more calories in absorbing and digesting food in the morning than in the evening.

Thermic effect of food (TEF) is a fancy name for the energy used up in the process of digesting and absorbing a meal. A study published in the *American Journal of Clinical Nutrition* found that TEF is higher in the morning than in the evening. Volunteers were given an identical 544-calorie meal at one of three times. In subjects fed at 9 a.m., TEF increased by 16 percent; in those fed at 5 p.m., TEF increased by 13.5 percent; and in those fed at 1 a.m., TEF increased by only 11 percent. So it's clear that we burn more calories in the morning.

However, according to surveys, more than 20 percent of Americans skip breakfast most days. Those who do eat breakfast too often choose sugary breakfast cereals, donuts, and baked goods that fail to provide sustained energy and balanced nutrition. A University of Massachusetts study found that those who regularly skip breakfast are 4.5 times more likely to be overweight than those who eat breakfast most mornings. This is probably because those who skip breakfast wind up eating more calories later in the day when activity levels and the body's metabolic rate are lower.

Also most men and women who skip breakfast eat a very large dinner. A study from the University of Texas, El Paso, found that the fewer calories subjects ate early in the day, the more total calories they ate over the course of the day. Overeating at any time of day encourages fat storage because more calories are taken in than are burned to meet energy needs, but overeating is worse in the evening because our body temperature is decreasing at this time, so fewer food calories are turned into body heat. By not skipping breakfast you will be less likely to overeat at supper and therefore you will be less likely to store excess calories as body fat.

The reason I recommend a breakfast of at least 250 calories is that it takes this much energy to replace the energy lost during the overnight fast and to fuel your body and mind for optimal functioning in the morning. Putting this nutrient timing method into practice is easy. If you're not currently eating breakfast, start eating it every day. If you do eat breakfast and your typical breakfast consists of a muffin and coffee, switch to breakfast choices that are more wholesome and substantial. On the next page are three examples of wholesome breakfast menus that provide at least 250 calories. See the four-week meal plan in Appendix B for other examples.

Nutrient Timing Tip #2: Keep your energy level consistent throughout the day with healthy snacks.

Unless you've been living under a rock, you have heard that eating snacks—or "grazing" throughout the day—is a good idea. While some dietary maxims have little evidence to support them, this one does. A study published in the *British Medical Journal* found that those who ate most frequently (five or more times a day) were thinner and had lower cholesterol and triglyceride levels than those who ate least often. The reason seems to be that more frequent eating reduces appetite, so you eat less at meals and consume fewer total calories throughout the day; and eating more frequently keeps your energy supply more consistent throughout the day, so you also tend to be more active.

However, other research has shown a link between frequent snacking and

BREAKFAST 1	BREAKFAST 2	BREAKFAST 3
½ cup old-fashioned oatmeal with sliced banana and a pinch of brown sugar	Scrambled egg whites (¾ cup) with mushrooms, spinach, onions, and diced tomatoes	1 cup Grape Nuts Flakes cereal with 8 ounces skim milk and ½ cup fresh blueberries
8 ounces orange juice	Whole-grain toast (1 slice) with 100% fruit spread	8 ounces orange juice
	Coffee	
430 calories	250 calories	350 calories

overeating. As you might expect, it is the quality of the snacks (and the meals they fall between) that makes the difference. Eating two or three snacks a day between meals won't automatically help you get leaner. Snacking will help only if the snacks satisfy your hunger without adding a huge number of calories to your total intake for the day. Naturally, the best snacks are those that have a relatively low caloric density, such as fruits and vegetables and whole-grain foods that are low in fat and sugar.

Most of us snack to some degree, but we do so spontaneously rather than conscientiously. Spontaneous snacking is eating a donut at the office only an hour after eating breakfast just because a coworker happens to arrive with a box of Krispy Kremes. Conscientious snacking is eating healthy snacks at least two hours after the last meal to keep your energy level high and your appetite at bay. If you are currently a spontaneous snacker, become a conscientious snacker during Phase II of the Lean Look program. Make a list of healthy snack foods you like, make sure to pick them up whenever you buy groceries, and have them available at the right times and places.

As with any new habit, becoming a conscientious snacker requires practice. It may take some time before you find snacks that are both healthy and satisfying enough to eliminate cravings for less wholesome choices, and it will take some planning ahead to have snacks available when and where you need them. You might find that it's easier to build this habit one snack at a time. For example, start by adding a midmorning snack to your schedule for a week or ten days. Once that's going well, add a midafternoon snack. And when that seems natural, add an evening protein snack (see Nutrient Timing Tip #7). Try to eat a variety of healthy snacks rather than having the same one or two snacks every time. Varying your snacks will help you achieve balanced nutrition, as no single food can supply everything your body needs.

You will find that snacking leaves you less hungry at mealtime. Reduce the size of your meals accordingly! If you add snacks (even if they're healthy snacks) to your daily eating schedule and continue to eat large meals out of habit instead of hunger, you won't get any leaner.

Nutrient Timing Tip #3: Bounce back faster after workouts with smart recovery nutrition.

If you work out—and on the Lean Look program you are, of course, working out six days a week—one of your daily meals or snacks should be taken within one hour of completing your workout. For example, if you exercise first thing in the morning, you should eat your breakfast within an hour of completing your workout. Again, this practice is in line with the principle of concentrating your caloric intake during times when your body needs energy most. The hour that immediately follows any period of strenuous activity is the time

---

10 HEALTHY SNACKS

1. Low-fat fruit-flavored yogurt (8 ounces)
2. Cashews or other nuts (1 palm)
3. Fresh fruit
4. Dried fruit (½ cup)
5. Carrot sticks and peanut butter (4–6 sticks)
6. Applesauce (½ cup)
7. Celery sticks dipped in low-fat ranch dressing
8. Fruit smoothies (Quick recipe: Blend 8 ounces orange juice, 1 whole banana, 1 cup frozen strawberries, and 4–6 ice cubes in a blender.)
9. Trail mix (peanuts, sunflower seeds, and raisins (1 palm)
10. 2-3 slices of smoked turkey

when your body needs energy most. Research shows that calories consumed within this window are put to excellent use: Protein is used to repair the microscopic damage to muscle tissue that occurs during workouts; carbohydrates are used to replenish your muscle and liver with glycogen (the muscles' main fuel source during intense workouts); and fats are used to meet immediate energy needs. It's also important to consume fluids within this window to replace body fluids lost through sweating during the workout.

Unfortunately, most exercisers scrupulously avoid taking in any kind of nutrition beyond water immediately after workouts. Intuition tells them that there are two ways to get rid of fat: exercising and not eating. So why not combine the two? Even worse, many so-called fitness experts who ought to know better explicitly promote this misguided practice. I don't know where they get this notion, but I do know that it's completely wrong: it's precisely those who avoid eating during the 60 minutes following exercise who wind up storing more fat—and building less muscle.

Muscle cells are highly insulin-sensitive immediately after exercise. Insulin is usually thought of as a fat-storing hormone, but it is also the most powerful muscle-fueling and muscle-building hormone. When you take in carbs and protein right after exercise, insulin will deliver these nutrients straight to the muscles to replenish their fuel stores and build new muscle tissue. If you wait two hours after exercising to consume the same nutrients, the carbs will more likely be converted to fat and the protein will not be usable.

These differences can add up over time. A Japanese study found that when animals were fed right after exercise versus four hours later, muscle weight was higher by 6 percent in the group fed immediately. The study also reported that abdominal fat was 24 percent lower in this group. The researchers concluded that the consumption of nutrients after exercise may contribute to an increase in muscle mass and a decrease in adipose tissue.

Similar results have been found in human studies. In a study reported in the *Journal of Physiology*, while participating in a 12-week strength-training program, subjects were given a carbohydrate-protein supplement either immediately after exercise or two hours later. The authors reported that when a carbohydrate-protein mixture was given immediately after each exercise session, muscle size increased 8 percent and strength improved 15 percent. When the supplement was given two hours later, there was no muscle growth or improvement in strength.

Another advantage of consuming carbs and protein immediately after exercise is that by increasing circulating insulin, you reduce circulating cortisol. After exercise, cortisol levels are very high. The main job of cortisol at this time is to break down muscle proteins for energy. This process gets in the way of repairing and building the muscles. Increasing insulin after exercise by eating carbs and protein is an important way to limit post-workout muscle protein breakdown and enhance muscle repair and building.

The ideal post-workout snack has plenty of carbs, a moderate amount of protein (a 4:1 ratio of carbs to protein is ideal), and a small amount of fat. (The timing issue is not as important with fats.) Examples of good post-workout snacks are toast with reduced-fat peanut butter, energy bars, and trail mix, washed down with water or 100 percent fruit juice. Since many of us are not particularly hungry during the first hour after a workout, specially formulated post-workout recovery drink mixes are another good option, because they are easy to get down even when you're not hungry and they provide the carbs, protein, and water you need in one fell swoop. The chart that follows lists recommended energy bars and performance recovery drinks. You can find such products at many bike shops and at nutritional supplement stores, including GNC.

Recommended Energy Bars	Recommended Performance Recovery Drinks
Balance Bar	Clif Shot Recovery®
ClifBar	Cytomax Recovery®
Detour	EAS Race Recovery
Peak Bar®	Endurox R⁴
PowerBar	PowerBar Performance Recovery
	Ultragen RS Recovery Drink

Nutrient Timing Tip #4: Prevent overeating at meals by eating appetite-spoiling appetizers.

Have you ever wondered what makes you feel full when you eat? Scientists have learned that satiety (the scientific word for the feeling of fullness) is caused primarily by the activation of hormonelike peptides (or protein fragments) that are produced in the gut in response to the presence of food. The three most important satiety peptides are known by the acronyms CCK, PYY, and GLP-1.

CCK was discovered first, in the 1970s. CCK is released in the small intestine when fats and proteins from a recent meal enter the duodenum. A rise in blood levels of CCK triggers the release of digestive enzymes from the pancreas and the delivery of bile from the gallbladder.

There are three mechanisms by which CCK produces satiety. It acts on nerves in the lining of your stomach that tell your brain your stomach is full; it slows the movement of food from your stomach so you feel full longer; and it sends a signal to the appetite control center in the brain resulting in cessation of the desire to eat.

The two other major satiety peptides, PYY and GLP-1, discovered more recently, act in similar ways. Interestingly, it is not food in general that causes these peptides to become activated, resulting in the feeling of fullness. Scientists have found that there are certain nutrients within foods that have a powerful stimulating effect on satiety peptides. Oleic acid, a type of fat, has the strongest stimulating effect on CCK. Certain compounds in milk protein and soy protein have the most potent stimulating effect on PYY. And oligofructose, a type of fiber, has the greatest stimulating effect on GLP-1.

Research has shown that foods containing high levels of one or more of these nutrients produce more of a sense of fullness per calorie than do the nutrients in other foods. What's more, it has also been shown that eating a small portion of such foods as appetizers before a meal significantly reduces subsequent eating during the meal. As a result men and women eat fewer total calories when a meal is preceded by one of these appetizers than when the meal is eaten alone.

Olive oil, avocados, and macadamia nuts have high levels of oleic acid. Wheat, tomatoes, and asparagus have high levels of oligofructose. Good sources of milk proteins include skim milk, low-fat or nonfat yogurt, and low-fat cheese. Soy proteins are found in all foods made from soy, including soy milk, soybeans, and tofu. To reduce your total calorie intake at meals (mainly dinner), eat a small appetizer containing one or more of these foods before you dig into your main meal. Take advantage of the fullness resulting from the appetizer by serving yourself smaller-than-normal portions. Washing down your appetizer with a glass of water or another noncaloric beverage will enhance the effect, because fluid distends the stomach, and stomach distension also activates CCK. The box that follows provides several examples of recommended appetite-spoiling appetizers.

APPETITE-SPOILING APPETIZERS

Garden salad (1 cup greens) with tomatoes, avocado, and olive oil-based dressing and 8 ounces water

Whole wheat crackers (3–4 crackers) with low-fat Cheddar cheese and 8 ounces water

Steamed asparagus (4–6 spears) drizzled with olive oil-based salad dressing and 8 ounces water

Edamame (steamed soybeans) — ½ cup

Glass of skim milk or soy milk (8 ounces)

Nutrient Timing Tip #5: Fuel stronger workouts with the right pre-workout meals.

At no other time during the day does your body use energy more than it does during a workout. Naturally you cannot and need not eat during a workout to provide this energy. Rather, it's the food energy you get from your last meal before the workout (stored energy) that will fuel it. Eating the right kinds of food at the right time before working out will help you to perform better in the workout and consequently get better results from it.

The first rule is not to work out on a full stomach. Blood flow is diverted to your visceral area during peak digestion, taking blood away from your muscles and compromising your workout performance. Working out on a full stomach is often also a recipe for gastrointestinal distress, especially if you're running. Your last full meal should be eaten at least two hours before your workout. It's okay to have a small, easily digested snack such as a piece of fruit or an 8-ounce tub of low-fat fruit-flavored yogurt up to 30 minutes before the workout. It may take some trial and error to determine the types, size, and timing of pre-workout snacks you can consume without experiencing stomach discomfort during a workout.

On the other hand, your workout probably should not follow your last full meal by more than four hours. If it does, your blood glucose and liver glycogen levels will be on their way down and you may feel sluggish. Many individuals find it most convenient to work out first thing in the morning, before they have a chance to eat. In this case, your best alternative to a pre-workout meal is to consume a carbohydrate sports drink during the workout (see Nutrient Timing Tip #8).

Be sure to consume high-carbohydrate foods (whole-grain breakfast cereals, old-fashioned oatmeal, fruit, whole-grain bread, yogurt, whole-wheat pasta) in your pre-workout meal. Recently consumed carbohydrates are the most readily available source of energy during exercise. If your pre-workout meal falls two to four hours before your workout, as it should, be sure to consume a meal with a low to moderate glycemic index. The glycemic index (GI) is a measure of how quickly the carbs in a meal enter your bloodstream. High GI meals provide fast energy that doesn't last too long. Moderate to low GI meals provide energy that comes on more slowly but lasts longer. The simplest way to ensure that your meal is in the range of moderate to low GI is to eat carbohydrate with some fat and protein, because fat and protein slow the absorption of carbohydrate. The box provides five examples of good pre-workout meals.

RECOMMENDED PRE-WORKOUT MEALS

Whole-grain breakfast cereal with skim milk
Grilled chicken Caesar salad plus 8 ounces 100 percent apple juice
Turkey sandwich with tomato and lettuce on whole-wheat bread
Stir-fried chicken and vegetables over brown rice
Whole-wheat spaghetti with tomato and vegetable sauce

Nutrient Timing Tip #6: Prevent overeating at meals by eating slowly.

Generally speaking, the faster we eat, the more we eat. When we wolf down our food instead of pacing ourselves and relishing our meals, chances are we will consume a larger number of calories than we need to satisfy our hunger. The reason is that there is a delay between the time food reaches our stomach and the time our appetite control mechanism is able to give our brain the signals needed to produce an actual feeling of fullness. Also when we eat quickly we are less likely to pay attention to this feeling of fullness.

The benefits of eating slowly were demonstrated in a study of 30 normal-weight women conducted by researchers at the University of Rhode Island. On two separate occasions they were instructed to eat the same pasta meal with water, consuming as much as they liked. But on one occasion they were told to eat as quickly as possible, while on the other occasion they were told to eat slowly and put down their fork between bites. The results showed that the women ate 67 fewer calories, on average, when they ate slowly, yet they remained full longer after eating slowly. Part of the reason was that they drank significantly more water when eating slowly.

Slowing down your eating is easy in principle, but it requires self-awareness to make it a habit that sticks. At first you might want to time your meals. Start by timing how long it takes you to eat a meal at your normal eating rate. Add 50 percent to this time and in subsequent meals put yourself on the clock, stretching out your eating time to match this new goal. Actually putting down your fork between bites is a trick that some dietitians teach their clients as a way to slow down their eating. I also find that it helps to sit for meals instead of standing, as too many of us do too often. Sitting encourages a more leisurely approach to the meal.

Conversation is another factor that slows down eating. After all, you can't talk and eat at the same time (or shouldn't!). In this regard, sharing meals with others is better than eating alone.

Nutrient Timing Tip #7: Build muscle overnight with a bedtime protein snack.

Growth hormone, as the name implies, is a potent muscle-building hormone in the human body. Circulating levels of growth hormone follow a circadian rhythm, peaking while you sleep and ebbing in the morning. This is important information for those who are trying to add lean muscle mass as part of an effort to get leaner. High levels of circulating growth hormone are not sufficient for muscle building. There must also be an adequate supply of amino acids with which to build muscle proteins. Eating a small, high-protein snack

PHASE II

before going to bed is the perfect way to provide these raw materials, allowing your body to become a little leaner while you dream. The box that follows provides some good examples of high-protein snacks you can eat before going to bed.

HIGH-PROTEIN BEDTIME SNACKS

Low-fat fruit-flavored yogurt (8-ounce tub)

Powdered whey protein drink mix (one serving)
(Examples: Designer Whey Protein Blast, GNC Pro Performance® 100% Whey Protein, Optimum Nutrition Classic Whey®, CytoSport Complete Whey Protein)

Rolled smoked turkey slices (3–4)

Glass of skim milk or soy milk (8 ounces)

Protein bar (½–1 bar)
(Examples: Detour, Met-Rx Protein Plus, Worldwide Sport Nutrition Pure Protein, Muscle Sandwich)

Nutrient Timing Tip #8: Fuel stronger workouts with sports drinks.

Anything you can do to enhance your performance in workouts will enhance the benefits you get from them, including the benefits of muscle toning and fat burning that will make you leaner. An important way to boost your workout performance nutritionally is by using a sports drink during workouts.

Most nonathletes consume either plain water or nothing at all during workouts. Water is better than nothing at all because it counteracts the reduction in blood volume that results from heavy sweating. Drinking water allows your heart to pump more blood and thereby send more oxygen to your muscles with each contraction, which in turn helps you to maintain a higher work level.

However, sports drinks such as Gatorade and Accelerade actually hydrate better than water because they contain sodium and carbohydrates, like your blood itself, and consequently maintain fluid balance in the blood and cells

POPULAR SPORTS DRINKS

Accelerade

Cytomax Ready-to-Drink

Gatorade Endurance Formula

Powerade

PHASE II

better. The carbohydrates in sports drinks also provide fast energy for your working muscles, enabling you to exercise at a higher intensity level (hence burn more fat and stimulate more muscle growth). Using a sports drink during exercise is especially beneficial if you work out first thing in the morning, before you've had a chance to eat anything. Your body is more glycogen depleted first thing in the morning than at any other time of day. Using a sports drink during your morning workout will help counteract this limitation.

The typical sports drink contains a fairly high amount of sugar—about half as much as the average soft drink. For this reason many sugar-conscious men and women try to steer clear of sports drinks, but there is no need to worry. During vigorous exercise your muscles essentially run on sugar. The sugars you consume in a sports drink during exercise are delivered straight to your muscles, where they are immediately converted to energy that enhances your workout performance. The ultimate result is that you get a better workout and enhanced benefits from the workout, including increased fat loss. Thus the effect of consuming sugars in a sports drink during exercise is precisely the opposite of the effect of consuming sugars in a soft drink while at rest. When you consume a large amount of sugar while inactive, most of these sugars are converted to fat and stored in adipose tissue.

Even many diabetics are able to benefit from using sports drinks during exercise, as the stress of exercise causes the body to strictly regulate blood sugar levels, thus preventing dangerous spikes or drops in blood sugar. However, some diabetics cannot safely consume sports drinks during exercise, so if you are diabetic, consult your doctor before using a sports drink in any workout.

Most sports drinks do not contain protein, but a growing number of the newer ones, including Accelerade, do. The reason is that recent research has shown that the addition of a small amount of protein to a sports drink boosts energy levels even more, reduces muscle tissue breakdown during the workout, and accelerates muscle protein building after the workout.

Have a bottle of sports drink handy during each workout. Take a swig every few minutes, according to your thirst, during the active recovery periods between cardio intervals and between exercises in your resistance exercise circuits.

RIGHT ON SCHEDULE

By incorporating these eight nutrient timing tips into your daily schedule during Phase II of the Lean Look program you will become leaner without cutting any additional calories. Exactly how you incorporate these nutrient timing tips depends on your lifestyle and certain preferences. For example, if you work a swing shift you won't eat on exactly the same schedule as a nine-to-fiver. The following charts present the first two days of the four-week meal plan that appears in Appendix B, modified to incorporate the nutrient timing practices. Day 1 is for a person who works out first thing in the morning. Day 2 is for a person who works out after work. Use these examples as a template and modify them to fit your needs and preferences. **Remember,** *eat slowly!*

Transitioning from your current eating schedule to this one might not be easy. But with a little discipline and a dash of determination you can do it. One of my current clients is Carol, a fifty-six-year-old retired schoolteacher and administrator who came to me after gaining 15 pounds in three years due to menopause. When I analyzed Carol's eating patterns I saw that she was stuck on the eating patterns she had grown accustomed to during her thirty-five-year career, but this kind of eating was not appropriate for her current leisurely retirement schedule. Specifically, while she was focused on work Carol was used to more or less starving herself until midafternoon, and then more than making up for lost time with a big late lunch and a big late dinner.

I encouraged Carol to change her eating schedule by eating early and often throughout the day and minding her portions at each sitting. She gave me some resistance—after all, she had spent thirty-five years giving instruction, not receiving it—but she gave it a try and after making a few adjustments to accommodate her preferences she found that nutrient timing really worked for her. She lowered her body fat percentage from 25 to 22 percent in the twelve weeks I was working with her—enough to make a dramatic difference in how she looked and felt. If Carol can make the switch to nutrient timing, you can too!

Day 1	
7:00 A.M. Workout	Cardio Workout (with Accelerade)
8:00 A.M. Breakfast/post-workout nutrition	Whole-wheat pancakes, Reduced-fat yogurt Diced fruit
10:00 A.M. Morning snack	Apple
12:00 Lunch	Mixed salad greens Chicken fajitas Apple
3:00 P.M. Afternoon snack	Whole-wheat toast
6:00 P.M. Appetizer	Light Cheddar cheese Water
6:15 P.M. Dinner	Wole-wheat pasta Tomato meat sauce Vegetable Salad Low-fat dressing
8:30 P.M. Evening snack	Powdered whey protein drink

Day 2

7:00 A.M. Breakfast	Reduced-fat yogurt Frozen berries Bran muffin
10:00 A.M. Morning snack	Peach
12:00 Lunch	Cheese pizza with whole-wheat crust Raw veggies with low-fat ranch dressing
3:00 P.M. Afternoon snack	Trail mix
5:30 P.M. Workout	Cardio workout (Gatorade Endurance Formula)
6:30 P.M. Appetizer	Edamame
6:45 P.M. Dinner/post-workout nutrition	Sweet 'n' sour chicken stir-fry with red peppers, broccoli, onions, mushrooms, and pineapple
8:30 P.M. Evening snack	Glass of soy milk

CHAPTER 10

Resistance Exercise: Strength Building

When you think about strength, you might get a mental picture of those Goliaths you see tossing monster truck tires around on ESPN2, competing for the title of "World's Strongest Man." These guys were born strong, and they spend hours each day training to become stronger. But you can benefit from strength training even if you don't have any interest in pulling tractor-trailer semis at the end of a tether. In fact, it could be a matter of complete indifference to you how strong you are, and it would still behoove you to do strength-building workouts.

The reason is that strength-building workouts also help you become leaner. As I mentioned earlier, there are several distinct types of resistance workouts you can do. Cycling through at least a few of them is better than doing any one of them exclusively all the time. And strength-building workouts are one type of resistance workout that should definitely have a place in this rotation. The development of your muscles can contribute to your becoming leaner directly, by growing, and indirectly, by burning more calories throughout the day (and the more they grow, the more calories they burn). Muscles become stronger primarily by becoming larger; individual muscle fibers become thicker, increasing the amount of resistance each can overcome when contracting. So by training to become stronger you develop fuller muscles and become leaner in direct and indirect ways.

It is not necessary to become as strong as a circus strong man or as pumped up as a bodybuilder to get visible results from strength-building workouts and to see a measurable difference in your body fat measurements. Very few of us are capable of getting anywhere near as strong or pumped up as these people anyway. It takes rare genes and thousands of hours in the gym. But with average genes and manageable workouts you can achieve a modest increase in muscle fullness that will subtly reshape your body to give you a more athletic appearance without making you larger. And even if you are not interested in strength, I think you will also come to appreciate the boost you get from doing strength-building workouts, especially on moving day!

When I introduce them to the type of training you will do in this phase of the Lean Look program, many of my female clients express fears of "bulking up," but they all find that these exercises do no such thing. A typical case is Jen, who was thirty-three years old and a new mother working as an account executive when she first came to my facility. Jen's goal was to lose her pregnancy weight plus 15 pounds—a goal I quickly translated into body fat percentage terms for her. Her diet was solid and needed only a few minor adjustments. She had done cardio exercise all her life, on the same equipment (bike and treadmill), but she had avoided lifting weights because (a) she was afraid she'd get big and bulky and (b) she didn't know how to lift weights correctly. She was intimidated in the gym by all the "super-fit" women, although she admired their physiques and wanted to be in the kind of shape they were in.

I started from the beginning with Jen, showing her how to use each piece of resistance-training equipment and teaching her proper form in a wide variety of exercises. I designed a training program for her that included as much resistance exercise as it did cardio work and I answered all of her questions. Then she was on her own. At last report she had lost all 12 pounds of her pregnancy weight plus 3 pounds of her pre-pregnancy weight, and no, she had not bulked up.

In Phase II of the Lean Look program the emphasis of your resistance workouts moves from muscle balancing to strength building with workouts based on 24 new exercises that are excellent strength builders. The overall goal—becoming leaner—remains unchanged. The switch in training is just a way of achieving greater leanness faster. The muscle-balancing resistance workouts of Phase I got your muscles accustomed to this type of exercise, prepared them for more challenging resistance workouts, and stimulated some initial gains in muscle tone. The strength-building resistance workouts you do in Phase II simply piggyback on the progress you made during Phase I.

A resistance workout designed to build strength must have two features. First, it should include some multi-joint exercises that involve the largest muscles of the body working cooperatively. In other words, it should involve some of the body's strongest movements. One example is the Sumo Squat (page 149), which simultaneously recruits the glutes, hamstrings, and back—three of the human body's largest and strongest muscle groups. This sort of exercise is quite different from the typical muscle-balancing exercise, which isolates individual muscle groups and pays special attention to the body's most neglected muscles.

The second essential quality of a strength-building resistance workout is increased resistance—that is, it involves amounts of resistance that are relatively close to the maximum amount you are able to lift for a given movement. When competitive weight lifters do strength-building workouts, they usually select weights equal to the maximum amount they can lift two to six times. Since the resistance workouts in the Lean Look program are designed as circuits with minimal rest between exercises, I will ask you to select loads you can lift 10 times with perfect form. The plus-one rule still applies, so you should complete that tenth repetition feeling as though you could squeeze out one more if you put all you have into it.

You will continue to do three resistance workouts per week throughout Phase II. Each week your first and third resistance workouts will be strength-building circuits. Your second resistance workout each week will be a muscle-balancing workout just like the workouts you did in Phase I, because it's important to maintain muscle balance even as you work on building strength.

Your strength-building resistance workouts will have the same basic structure as the workouts you did in Phase I. Choose 9 resistance exercises to do in each workout, if you're following the beginner schedule; choose 12 if you're following the advanced schedule. Exercises are also classified according to which area of the body they target: legs, core, and upper body. For example, a strength-building resistance workout with three exercises per body area would look like this: Leg exercise #1, Core exercise #1, Upper body exercise #1, Leg exercise #2, Core exercise #2, Upper body exercise #2, Leg exercise #3, Core exercise #3, Upper body exercise #3. Try to avoid choosing multiple exercises that target the same muscles within a given area of the body.

Different exercises require different equipment (while a few weight-bearing exercises require none). With 24 strength-building exercises to choose from, you can easily put together a complete workout that does not involve one of the major equipment items (dumbbells or cable resistance). In the final section of the chapter I will present ready-made beginner and advanced strength-building resistance workouts involving either dumbbells and an exercise bench only or cable resistance and a stability ball only. Choose the appropriate ready-made strength-building resistance workout to follow throughout Phase II if you don't have access to all of the equipment or if you simply don't feel like designing your own workouts drawing from the pool of 24 strength-building exercises.

Don't rest between exercises. Warm up for each resistance workout by doing a few of the dynamic warm-up exercises on page 64.

STRENGTH-BUILDING RESISTANCE EXERCISES

These 24 exercises have been selected based on their effectiveness as strength builders. There are 8 exercises each for the legs, core (abs and back), and upper body.

LEG EXERCISES

Following are 8 strength-building resistance exercises for the legs.

Sumo Squat

MUSCLES TARGETED: hamstrings, quadriceps, buttocks

EQUIPMENT REQUIRED: dumbbell

Stand in a broad stance with your feet angled slightly outward. Grasp a heavy dumbbell with both hands and your arms fully extended toward the floor in front of your body. Set your core. Maintaining a neutral spinal posture, squat down deeply. Pause briefly at the bottom of the movement and then stand fully upright by powerfully contracting your hamstrings, buttocks, and lower back.

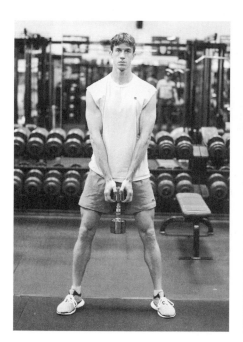
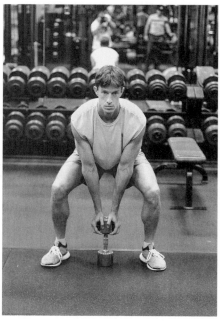

Single-Leg Squat with Stability Ball

MUSCLES TARGETED: quadriceps, hamstrings, hips, buttocks

EQUIPMENT REQUIRED: stability ball

Stand about 2 feet in front of a stability ball and rest your left foot on it. Set your core. Squat down as far as you can go without feeling unstable or straining your right knee, keeping your spine neutral and your hips even (don't let the unsupported hip "dip" toward the floor). Pause briefly at the bottom of the movement and then press back upright. After completing a full set, switch legs.

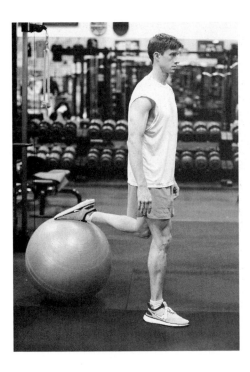
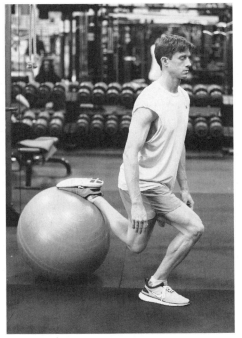

Squat with Dumbbells

MUSCLES TARGETED: quadriceps, hamstrings, buttocks

EQUIPMENT REQUIRED: dumbbells

Stand normally with your arms at your sides and a dumbbell in each hand. Set your core. Squat toward the floor until your thighs are parallel to it, or as far as you can comfortably go. Concentrate on keeping your weight on your heels and avoid arching your lower back. Now press powerfully back upright. As an alternative to dumbbells you can do this exercise with a weighted barbell braced against your upper back.

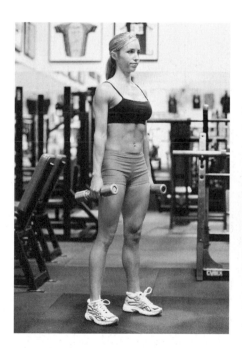
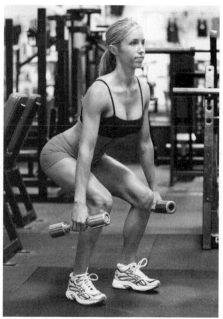

PHASE II

151

Forward Lunge

MUSCLES TARGETED: quadriceps, hamstrings, buttocks

EQUIPMENT REQUIRED: dumbbells

Stand with your feet placed at shoulder width and your toes forward. Hold a dumbbell in each hand with your arms extended toward the floor. Set your core. Take a large step forward with your right leg and dip down until your right thigh is parallel to the floor. Push off the floor with your right heel and return to the start position. Do a full set with your right leg, then switch to your left leg.

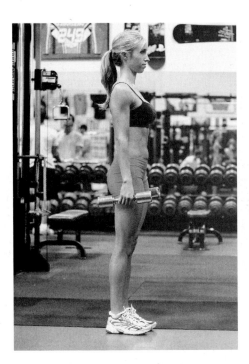
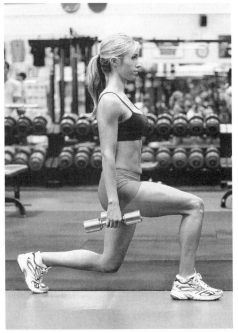

Split Squat

MUSCLES TARGETED: quadriceps, hamstrings, hips, buttocks

EQUIPMENT REQUIRED: dumbbells

Stand in a split stance, with your left foot half a pace in front of the right. Your left leg is straight and your left foot is flat on the ground. Your right leg is slightly bent and only the toes are in contact with the floor. Grasp a dumbbell in each hand with your arms at your sides. Set your core. Squat toward the floor until your left thigh is parallel to it, or as far as you can comfortably go. Keep your weight on your left heel and avoid rounding or arching your spine. Press back to a standing position. After completing a full set, reverse your stance and repeat the exercise.

PHASE II

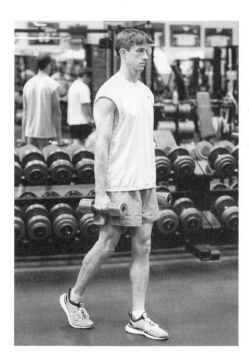
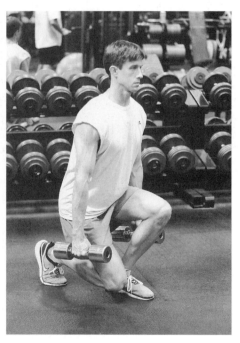

Stability Ball Leg Curl

MUSCLES TARGETED: hamstrings, buttocks

EQUIPMENT REQUIRED: stability ball

Lie faceup and place your heels together on top of a stability ball. Raise your pelvis so that your body forms a straight plank from head to toes. Set your core. Contract your glutes and hamstrings and roll the ball toward your buttocks. Pause briefly and return to the start position. Focus on keeping your pelvis from sagging toward the floor throughout this movement.

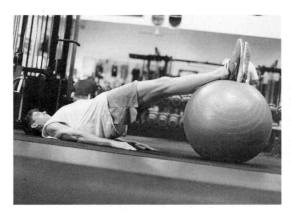 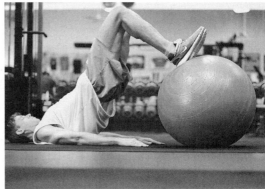

Weighted Heel Raise

MUSCLES TARGETED: calves

EQUIPMENT REQUIRED: dumbbells

Stand with your feet close together, your arms at your sides, and a dumbbell in each hand. Set your core. Contract your calf muscles and lift your heels as high off the floor as possible. Return to the starting position.

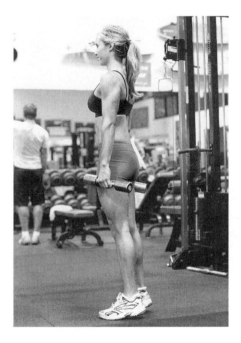 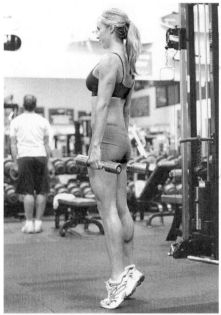

Supine Bridge Heel Raise

MUSCLES TARGETED: calves

EQUIPMENT REQUIRED: exercise bench or stability ball

Place your feet in a wide stance on the floor, rest your upper back, shoulders, and head on a bench or stability ball, and balance your weight in between. Your shins are at a right angle to the floor and your body is parallel to the floor from the knees to the neck. Set your core. Contract your calf muscles and raise your heels off the floor as high as possible. Pause for 1 second and return to the start position. After completing a full set, switch legs.

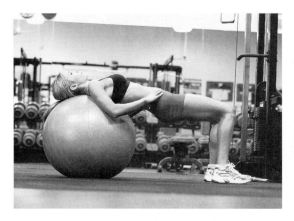 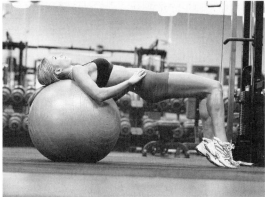

CORE EXERCISES

Following are 8 strength-building resistance exercises for the core (abs and back).

V-Up

MUSCLES TARGETED: outer abs

EQUIPMENT REQUIRED: none

Lie faceup with your legs fully extended and your arms fully outstretched behind you. Set your core. Contract your abdominal muscles and simultaneously lift your back and legs off the floor, trying to reach your toes with your fingers. You may find this exercise difficult to coordinate at first. If you have trouble getting the hang of it, do a modified V-Up with your knees bent.

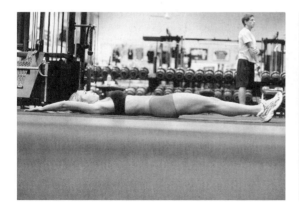 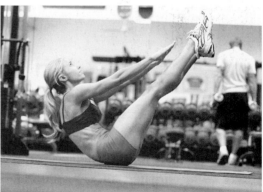

Weighted Stability Ball Crunch

MUSCLES TARGETED: outer abs

EQUIPMENT REQUIRED: stability ball, any type of weight

Perform this exercise exactly like the standard Stability Ball Crunch described on page 81, but instead of lacing your fingers behind your head, use both hands to brace some form of weight (dumbbell, weight plate, medicine ball) against your chest. If you do not have access to a useful form of weight, do the exercise with your arms extended straight overhead.

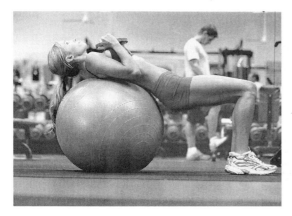 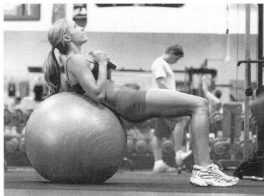

Chin-up

MUSCLES TARGETED: back

EQUIPMENT REQUIRED: chin-up bar

Begin hanging from a chin-up bar with an overhand grip on the bar and your hands positioned slightly farther than shoulder width apart. Set your core. Pull your body upward toward the bar until your chin is level with the bar. Pause briefly and slowly lower yourself back to the starting position.

If you cannot complete at least 8 chin-ups, do a modified chin-up: In order to do this exercise you need to have some sort of sturdy rod secured three to four feet above the floor. A broom handle laid across a pair of barstools will do the trick. Sit under the bar and grab it underhand with your hands positioned at shoulder width. Raise your hips up and form a straight line with your whole body. You are now "hanging" from the bar with only your heels touching the floor. Pull your chest to the bar and then return slowly to a hanging position.

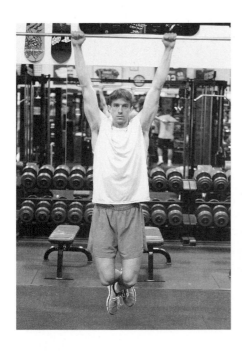
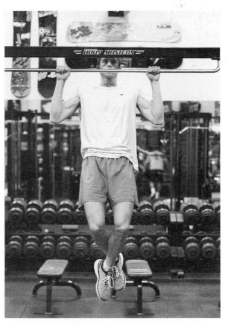

Bent-Over Cable Row

MUSCLES TARGETED: back

EQUIPMENT REQUIRED: cable resistance

Stand facing a cable pulley station in a split stance with your right foot positioned a step ahead of your left. Bend forward 30 degrees from the hips. With your left hand, grasp a handle affixed to a low attachment point. Begin with your arm fully extended toward the attachment point. Set your core. Contract the large muscles of your back and pull the handle toward the rib cage on the left side of your body. Pause briefly and return to the starting position. After completing a full set, reverse your stance and pull with your right arm.

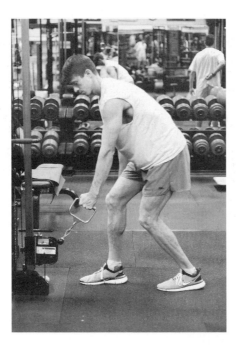
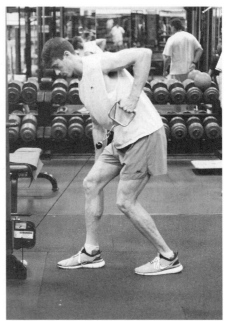

L-Over

MUSCLES TARGETED: deep abs, obliques

EQUIPMENT REQUIRED: none

Lie faceup with your arms resting at your sides and your palms flat on the floor. Extend your legs directly toward the ceiling, touch your feet together, and point your toes. Set your core. Keeping your big toes side-by-side, tip your legs 12 to 18 inches to the right by twisting at the hip, so that your right butt cheek comes off the floor. Fight the pull of gravity by maintaining stability with your abs and obliques. Pause for a moment, then return slowly to the starting position, again using your core muscles to control the movement. Repeat on the left side, and continue alternating from right to left until you have completed a full set.

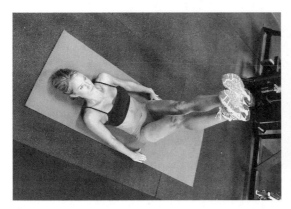
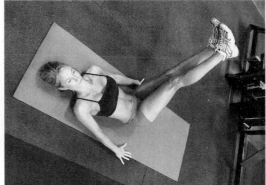

Crunch Twist

MUSCLES TARGETED: outer abs, obliques

EQUIPMENT REQUIRED: none

Lie faceup on a floor mat. Raise your head and upper shoulders off the mat just slightly and lace the fingers of both hands together behind your head for support, keeping your elbows wide. Begin with your knees bent 90 degrees, your thighs perpendicular to the floor, and your shins parallel to the floor. Set your core. Contract your stomach muscles and at the same time twist your torso to the right, so your left elbow moves toward your right knee. Pause at the height of the movement, then return to the start position, and repeat on the other side.

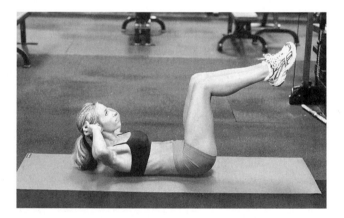

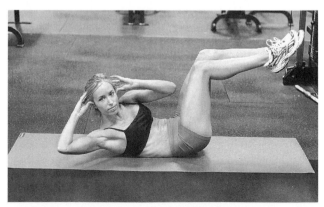

Reverse Crunch

MUSCLES TARGETED: lower abs

EQUIPMENT REQUIRED: none

Lie faceup on a comfortable surface. Raise your head and upper shoulders off the mat just slightly and lace the fingers of both hands together behind your head for support, keeping your elbows wide. Bend your knees 90 degrees and raise your feet an inch or two above the mat, as well. Set your core. Lift your knees in a smooth arc toward your head, while keeping the rest of your body still. When your knees are directly above your upper abdomen, pause briefly then reverse direction and lower your feet back toward the floor, but do not let them touch down. Maintain constant tension in your stomach muscles.

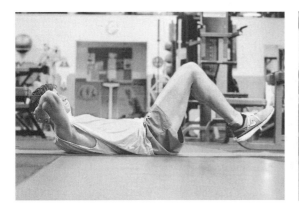 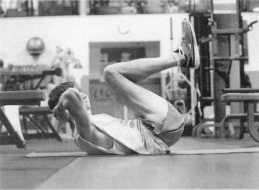

Stability Ball Back Extension

MUSCLES TARGETED: lower back

EQUIPMENT REQUIRED: stability ball

Lie facedown on a stability ball with the ball supporting your torso/upper thigh area and your toes in contact with the floor. Begin with your lower back muscles relaxed and your upper torso and arms angled toward the floor. Set your core. Now contract your lower back muscles and lift your upper torso and arms upward as far as you can. Pause briefly at the top of the movement and then relax again.

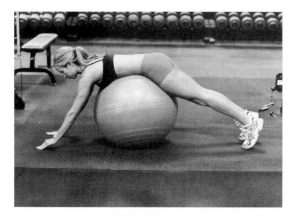 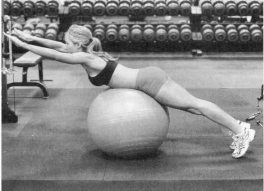

UPPER BODY EXERCISES

Following are 8 strength-building resistance exercises for the upper body (chest, shoulders, and arms).

Chest Dip

MUSCLES TARGETED: chest, triceps, rear shoulders

EQUIPMENT REQUIRED: exercise benches (2) or chairs (2)

Place two exercise benches or sturdy chairs 24 to 30 inches apart. Balance yourself between them on your palms with your legs outstretched and only your heels resting on the floor in front of you. Your arms should be straight and in line with your torso, with your fingers pointing ahead. Set your core. Lower your body toward the floor several inches by bending at the elbows and then press back upward to the start position.

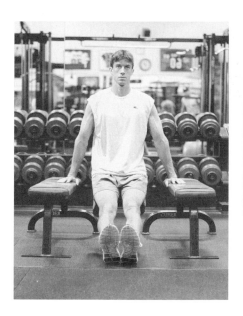 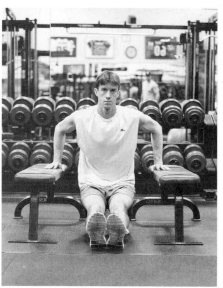

PHASE II

Standing Single-Arm Cable Flye

MUSCLES TARGETED: chest, rear shoulders

EQUIPMENT REQUIRED: cable resistance

Stand approximately 4 feet away from a door gym or cable pulley station with your right side facing it. Connect a handle to the high attachment point. Extend your right arm straight toward the door gym or cable pulley station and grasp the handle with your palm facing forward. Set your core. Keeping your arm extended, pull the handle away from the door gym or cable pulley station all the way across your chest. Pause and return to the starting position. After completing a full set, turn around and do the exercise with your left arm.

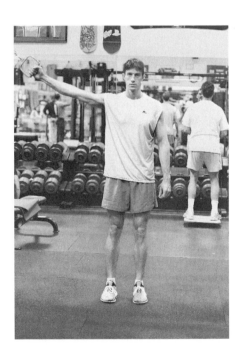 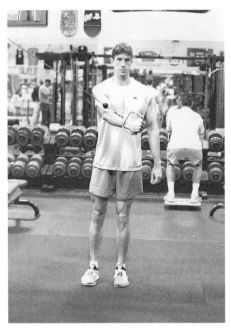

Alternating Shoulder Press

MUSCLES TARGETED: shoulders, triceps

EQUIPMENT REQUIRED: dumbbells

Stand normally with a dumbbell in each hand. Begin with your arms sharply bent so that the dumbbells are positioned just above each shoulder. Set your core. Press the dumbbell in your right hand straight overhead, pause briefly, and then lower it back toward your shoulder. Now do the same with the dumbbell in your left hand.

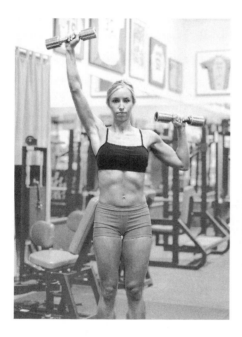
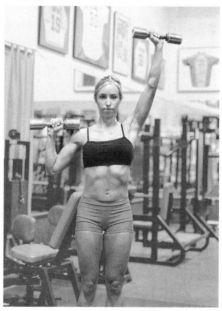

Stability Ball Triceps Press

MUSCLES TARGETED: triceps, upper back, chest

EQUIPMENT REQUIRED: stability ball

Assume a push-up position with your toes on the floor and your hands placed close together on a stability ball. Set your core. Bend your elbows and lower your chest toward the ball until you are within an inch of touching it, then press back to the starting position. This exercise is most challenging when you do it without bending forward at the waist. You can make it easier by moving your feet closer to the ball and bending at the waist.

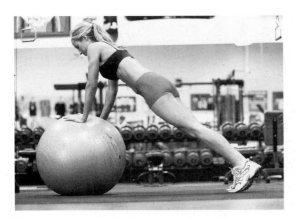
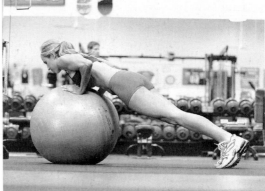

Biceps Curl

MUSCLES TARGETED: biceps

EQUIPMENT REQUIRED: dumbbells

Stand normally with your arms at your sides and a dumbbell in each hand. Begin with your palms facing in. Set your core. Keeping your upper arms locked in line with your body, bend your elbows fully and curl the dumbbells toward your shoulders and at the same time rotate your forearms outward. Pause when your elbows are fully flexed and then slowly lower the dumbbells.

PHASE II

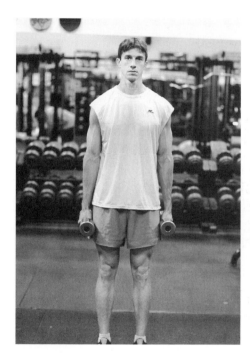
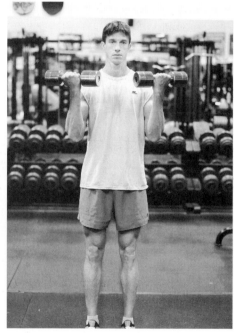

Cable Curl and Press

MUSCLES TARGETED: biceps, shoulders

EQUIPMENT REQUIRED: cable resistance

Stand facing a door gym or cable pulley station with a handle connected to a low attachment point. Begin with both arms relaxed at your sides and grasp the handle in your right hand, palm forward. Set your core. Contract your right biceps and curl the handle toward your collarbone. When your elbow is fully flexed, extend your right arm straight toward the ceiling while rotating your forearm so that your palm is once again facing the door gym or cable pulley station. Pause briefly with your arm straight upward and then reverse the previous movement in two steps. After completing a full set, repeat the exercise with your left arm.

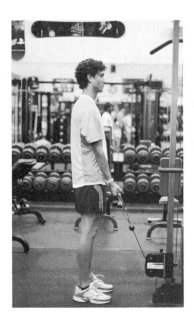 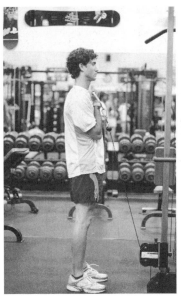 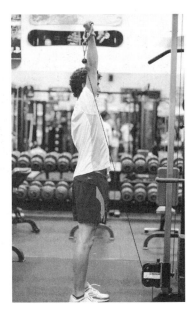

Triceps Press

MUSCLES TARGETED: triceps

EQUIPMENT REQUIRED: dumbbell

Stand normally with your right arm raised straight overhead and a dumbbell in your right hand. Set your core. Bend your elbow and lower the dumbbell behind your head. Go as far as you can without hitting yourself and then extend your arm again. After completing a full set, work your left arm.

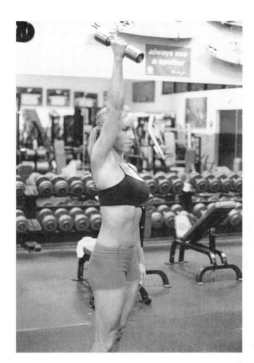 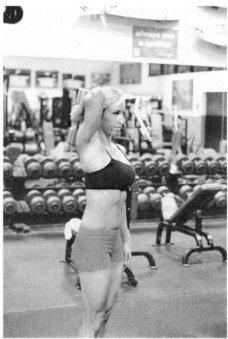

PHASE II

Bent-Over Cable Side Shoulder Raise

MUSCLES TARGETED: shoulders

EQUIPMENT REQUIRED: cable resistance

Stand in a wide stance with your knees slightly bent and your left side facing a door gym or cable pulley station with a handle connected to the low attachment point. Grasp the handle in your right hand using an underhand grip. Bend forward 45 degrees from the hips. Begin with your right arm extended toward the floor and the handle positioned directly underneath your left shoulder. Set your core. Now pull the handle outward and upward until your right arm is fully extended away from your body parallel to the floor. Pause briefly and return to the starting position. After completing a full set, reverse your position and work the left shoulder.

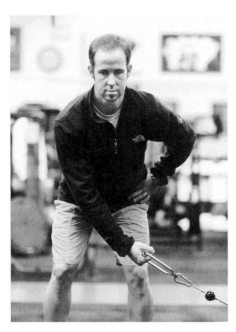 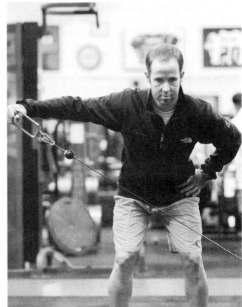

The following chart provide summary information about all 24 of the strength-building exercises presented in this chapter. Use this chart and the workout guidelines provided earlier on page 147 to design you own strength-building resistance workouts, or choose an appropriate ready-made workout from those provided in the next section.

SUMMARY OF STRENGTH-BUILDING RESISTANCE EXERCISES

EXERCISE	EQUIPMENT	MUSCLES TARGETED
LEG EXERCISES		
Sumo Squat	Dumbbell	Hamstrings, quadriceps, buttocks
Single-Leg Squat with Stability Ball	Stability ball	Quadriceps, hamstrings, hips, buttock
Squat with Dumbbells	Dumbbells	Hips, quadriceps, buttocks
Forward Lunge	Dumbbells	Hamstrings, quadriceps, buttocks
Split Squat	Dumbbells	Quadriceps, hamstrings, hips, buttocks
Stability Ball Leg Curl	Stability ball	Hamstrings, buttocks
Weighted Heel Raise	Dumbbells	Calves
Supine Bridge Heel Raise	Exercise bench or stability ball	Calves
CORE EXERCISES		
V-Up	None	Outer abs
Weighted Stability Ball Crunch	Stability ball, any type of weight	Outer abs
Chin-up	Chin-up bar	Back
Bent-Over Cable Row	Cable resistance	Back
L-Over	None	Deep abs, obliques
Crunch Twist	None	Outer abs, obliques

Reverse Crunch	None	Lower abs
Stability Ball Back Extension	Stability ball	Lower back

UPPER BODY EXERCISES

Chest Dip	Two exercise benches or two chairs	Chest, triceps, rear, shoulders
Standing Single-Arm Cable Flye	Cable resistance	Chest, rear shoulders
Alternating Shoulder Press	Dumbbells	Shoulders, triceps
Stability Ball Triceps Press	Stability ball	Triceps, upper back, chest
Biceps Curl	Dumbbell	Biceps
Cable Curl and Press	Cable resistance	Biceps, shoulders
Triceps Press	Dumbbell	Triceps
Bent-Over Cable Side Shoulder Raise	Cable resistance	Shoulders

READY-MADE STRENGTH-BUILDING RESISTANCE CIRCUITS

The charts that follow present ready-made strength-building resistance circuits for use in Phase II of the Lean Look program. There are two beginner circuits (consisting of 9 exercises) and two advanced circuits (consisting of 12 exercises). One of the beginner circuits and one of the advanced circuits require just a stability ball and cable resistance. The other beginner circuit and advanced circuit require only an exercise bench and dumbbells.

These ready-made circuits do not represent complete workouts. You will perform two to three complete circuits (i.e., you will repeat your chosen circuit two or three times) as prescribed in the Phase II resistance workout schedules provided at the end of the chapter.

BEGINNER STRENGTH-BUILDING RESISTANCE CIRCUIT #1 (9 EXERCISES)

Equipment: stability ball and cable resistance

Leg Exercise #1	Single-Leg Squat with Stability Ball (page 150)
Core Exercise #1	Weighted Stability Ball Crunch (page 158)
Upper Body Exercise #1	Standing Single-Arm Cable Flye (page 166)
Leg Exercise #2	Stability Ball Leg Curl (page 154)
Core Exercise #2	Bent-over Cable Row (page 160)
Upper Body Exercise #2	Stability Ball Triceps Press (page 168)
Leg Exercise #3	Supine Bridge Heel Raise (page 156)
Core Exercise #3	Stability Ball Back Extension (page 164)
Upper Body Exercise #3	Cable Curl and Press (page 170)

BEGINNER STRENGTH-BUILDING RESISTANCE CIRCUIT #2 (9 EXERCISES)

Equipment: exercise bench and dumbbells

Leg Exercise #1	Sumo Squat (page 149)
Core Exercise #1	V-Up (page 157)
Upper Body Exercise #1	Chest Dip (page 165)
Leg Exercise #2	Squat with Dumbbells (page 151)
Core Exercise #2	Chin-up (page 159)
Upper Body Exercise #2	Alternating Shoulder Press (page 167)
Leg Exercise #3	Weighted Heel Raise (page 155)
Core Exercise #3	L-Over (page 161)
Upper Body Exercise #3	Biceps Curl (page 169)

ADVANCED STRENGTH-BUILDING WORKOUT #1 (12 EXERCISES)

Equipment: stability ball and cable resistance

Leg Exercise #1	Single-Leg Squat with Stability Ball (page 150)
Core Exercise #1	Weighted Stability Ball Crunch (page 158)
Upper Body Exercise #1	Standing Single-Arm Cable Flye (page 166)
Leg Exercise #2	Stability Ball Leg Curl (page 154)
Core Exercise #2	Bent-over Cable Row (page 160)
Upper Body Exercise #2	Stability Ball Triceps Press (page 168)
Leg Exercise #3	Forward Lunge (page 152)
Core Exercise #3	Reverse Crunch (page 163)
Upper Body Exercise #3	Bent-over Cable Side Shoulder Raise (page 172)
Leg Exercise #4	Supine Bridge Heel Raise (page 156)
Core Exercise #4	Stability Ball Back Extension (page 164)
Upper Body Exercise #4	Cable Curl and Press (page 170)

ADVANCED STRENGTH-BUILDING WORKOUT #2 (12 EXERCISES)

Equipment: exercise bench and dumbbells

Leg Exercise #1	Sumo Squat (page 149)
Core Exercise #1	V-up (page 157)
Upper Body Exercise #1	Chest Dip (page 165)
Leg Exercise #2	Squat with Dumbbells (page 151)
Core Exercise #2	Chin-up (page 159)
Upper Body Exercise #2	Alternating Shoulder Press (page 167)
Leg Exercise #3	Split Squat (page 153)
Core Exercise #3	Crunch Twist (page 162)
Upper Body Exercise #3	Triceps Press (page 171)
Leg Exercise #4	Weighted Heel Raise (page 155)
Core Exercise #4	L-over (page 161)
Upper Body Exercise #4	Biceps Curl (page 169)

DETAILED PHASE II RESISTANCE WORKOUT SCHEDULES

Detailed Phase II resistance workout schedules for the beginner level and the advanced level appear on the following pages. Throughout this phase you will do strength-building resistance workouts as described in this chapter on Monday and Friday. On Wednesday you will continue to do a muscle-balancing resistance workout as you did throughout Phase I.

BEGINNER SCHEDULE

Wk #	Monday	Wednesday	Friday
5	Strength-Building Resistance Workout	Muscle-Balancing Resistance Workout	Strength-Building Resistance Workout
	Summary 2 circuits 9 exercises 21 minutes	Summary 2 circuits 9 exercises 21 minutes	Summary 2 circuits 9 exercises 21 minutes
	Workout:	Workout:	Workout:
	Warm-up	Warm-up	Warm-up
	2X Strength-Building Leg Exercise #1	2X Muscle-Balancing Leg Exercise #1	2X Strength-Building Leg Exercise #1
	Strength-Building Core Exercise #1	Muscle-Balancing Core Exercise #1	Strength-Building Core Exercise #1
	Strength-Building Upper Body Exercise #1	Muscle-Balancing Upper Body Exercise #1	Strength-Building Upper Body Exercise #1
	Strength-Building Leg Exercise #2	Muscle-Balancing Leg Exercise #2	Strength-Building Leg Exercise #2
	Strength-Building Core Exercise #2	Muscle-Balancing Core Exercise #2	Strength-Building Core Exercise #2
	Strength-Building Upper Body Exercise #2	Muscle-Balancing Upper Body Exercise #2	Strength-Building Upper Body Exercise #2
	Strength-Building Leg Exercise #3	Muscle-Balancing Leg Exercise #3	Strength-Building Leg Exercise #3

Wk #	Monday	Wednesday	Friday
5	Strength-Building Core Exercise #3	Muscle-Balancing Core Exercise #3	Strength-Building Core Exercise #3
	Strength-Building Upper Body Exercise #3	Muscle-Balancing Upper Body Exercise #3	Strength-Building Upper Body Exercise #3

Wk #	Monday	Wednesday	Friday
6	Strength-Building Resistance Workout	Muscle-Balancing Resistance Workout	Strength-Building Resistance Workout
	Summary 3 circuits 9 exercises 30 minutes	Summary 3 circuits 9 exercises 30 minutes	Summary 3 circuits 9 exercises 30 minutes
	Workout:	Workout:	Workout:
	Warm-up	Warm-up	Warm-up
	3X Strength-Building Leg Exercise #1	3X Muscle-Balancing Leg Exercise #1	3X Strength-Building Leg Exercise #1
	Strength-Building Core Exercise #1	Muscle-Balancing Core Exercise #1	Strength-Building Core Exercise #1
	Strength-Building Upper Body Exercise #1	Muscle-Balancing Upper Body Exercise #1	Strength-Building Upper Body Exercise #1
	Strength-Building Leg Exercise #2	Muscle-Balancing Leg Exercise #2	Strength-Building Leg Exercise #2
	Strength-Building Core Exercise #2	Muscle-Balancing Core Exercise #2	Strength-Building Core Exercise #2
	Strength-Building Upper Body Exercise #2	Muscle-Balancing Upper Body Exercise #2	Strength-Building Upper Body Exercise #2
	Strength-Building Leg Exercise #3	Muscle-Balancing Leg Exercise #3	Strength-Building Leg Exercise #3
	Strength-Building Core Exercise #3	Muscle-Balancing Core Exercise #3	Strength-Building Core Exercise #3
	Strength-Building Upper Body Exercise #3	Muscle-Balancing Upper Body Exercise #3	Strength-Building Upper Body Exercise #3

Wk #	Monday	Wednesday	Friday
7	Strength-Building Resistance Workout	Muscle-Balancing Resistance Workout	Strength-Building Resistance Workout
	Summary 3 circuits 9 exercises 30 minutes	Summary 3 circuits 9 exercises 30 minutes	Summary 3 circuits 9 exercises 30 minutes
	Workout:	Workout:	Workout:
	Warm-up	Warm-up	Warm-up
	3X Strength-Building Leg Exercise #1	3X Muscle-Balancing Leg Exercise #1	3X Strength-Building Leg Exercise #1
	Strength-Building Core Exercise #1	Muscle-Balancing Core Exercise #1	Strength-Building Core Exercise #1
	Strength-Building Upper Body Exercise #1	Muscle-Balancing Upper Body Exercise #1	Strength-Building Upper Body Exercise #1
	Strength-Building Leg Exercise #2	Muscle-Balancing Leg Exercise #2	Strength-Building Leg Exercise #2
	Strength-Building Core Exercise #2	Muscle-Balancing Core Exercise #2	Strength-Building Core Exercise #2
	Strength-Building Upper Body Exercise #2	Muscle-Balancing Upper Body Exercise #2	Strength-Building Upper Body Exercise #2
	Strength-Building Leg Exercise #3	Muscle-Balancing Leg Exercise #3	Strength-Building Leg Exercise #3
	Strength-Building Core Exercise #3	Muscle-Balancing Core Exercise #3	Strength-Building Core Exercise #3
	Strength-Building Upper Body Exercise #3	Muscle-Balancing Upper Body Exercise #3	Strength-Building Upper Body Exercise #3

Wk #	Monday	Wednesday	Friday
8	Strength-Building Resistance Workout	Muscle-Balance Resistance Workout	Strength-Building Resistance Workout
	Summary 2 circuits 9 exercises 21 minutes	Summary 2 circuits 9 exercises 21 minutes	Summary 2 circuits 9 exercises 21 minutes
	Workout:	Workout:	Workout:
	Warm-up	Warm-up	Warm-up

PHASE II

Wk #	Monday	Wednesday	Friday
8	2X Strength-Building Leg Exercise #1 Strength-Building Core Exercise #1 Strength-Building Upper Body Exercise #1 Strength-Building Leg Exercise #2 Strength-Building Core Exercise #2 Strength-Building Upper Body Exercise #2 Strength-Building Leg Exercise #3 Strength-Building Core Exercise #3 Strength-Building Upper Body Exercise #3	2X Muscle-Balancing Leg Exercise #1 Muscle-Balancing Core Exercise #1 Muscle-Balancing Upper Body Exercise #1 Muscle-Balancing Leg Exercise #2 Muscle-Balancing Core Exercise #2 Muscle-Balancing Upper Body Exercise #2 Muscle-Balancing Leg Exercise #3 Muscle-Balancing Core Exercise #3 Muscle-Balancing Upper Body Exercise #3	2X Strength-Building Leg Exercise #1 Strength-Building Core Exercise #1 Strength-Building Upper Body Exercise #1 Strength-Building Leg Exercise #2 Strength-Building Core Exercise #2 Strength-Building Upper Body Exercise #2 Strength-Building Leg Exercise #3 Strength-Building Core Exercise #3 Strength-Building Upper Body Exercise #3

ADVANCED SCHEDULE

Wk #	Monday	Wednesday	Friday
5	Strength-Building Resistance Workout	Muscle-Balancing Resistance Workout	Strength-Building Resistance Workout
	Summary 2 circuits 12 exercises 27 minutes	Summary 2 circuits 12 exercises 27 minutes	Summary 2 circuits 12 exercises 27 minutes
	Workout:	Workout:	Workout:
	Warm-up	Warm-up	Warm-up
	2X Strength-Building Leg Exercise #1	2X Muscle-Balancing Leg Exercise #1	2X Strength-Building Leg Exercise #1
	Strength-Building Core Exercise #1	Muscle-Balancing Core Exercise #1	Strength-Building Core Exercise #1
	Strength-Building Upper Body Exercise #1	Muscle-Balancing Upper Body Exercise #1	Strength-Building Upper Body Exercise #1
	Strength-Building Leg Exercise #2	Muscle-Balancing Leg Exercise #2	Strength-Building Leg Exercise #2
	Strength-Building Core Exercise #2	Muscle-Balancing Core Exercise #2	Strength-Building Core Exercise #2
	Strength-Building Upper Body Exercise #2	Muscle-Balancing Upper Body Exercise #2	Strength-Building Upper Body Exercise #2
	Strength-Building Leg Exercise #3	Muscle-Balancing Leg Exercise #3	Strength-Building Leg Exercise #3
	Strength-Building Core Exercise #3	Muscle-Balancing Core Exercise #3	Strength-Building Core Exercise #3
	Strength-Building Upper Body Exercise #3	Muscle-Balancing Upper Body Exercise #3	Strength-Building Upper Body Exercise #3
	Strength-Building Leg Exercise #4	Muscle-Balancing Leg Exercise #4	Strength-Building Leg Exercise #4
	Strength-Building Core Exercise #4	Muscle-Balancing Core Exercise #4	Strength-Building Core Exercise #4
	Strength-Building Upper Body Exercise #4	Muscle-Balancing Upper Body Exercise #4	Strength-Building Upper Body Exercise #4

PHASE II

Wk #	Monday	Wednesday	Friday
6	Strength-Building Resistance Workout	Muscle-Balancing Resistance Workout	Strength-Building Resistance Workout
	Summary 3 circuits 12 exercises 39 minutes	Summary 3 circuits 12 exercises 39 minutes	Summary 3 circuits 12 exercises 39 minutes
	Workout:	Workout:	Workout:
	Warm-up	Warm-up	Warm-up
	3X Strength-Building Leg Exercise #1	3X Muscle-Balancing Leg Exercise #1	3X Strength-Building Leg Exercise #1
	Strength-Building Core Exercise #1	Muscle-Balancing Core Exercise #1	Strength-Building Core Exercise #1
	Strength-Building Upper Body Exercise #1	Muscle-Balancing Upper Body Exercise #1	Strength-Building Upper Body Exercise #1
	Strength-Building Leg Exercise #2	Muscle-Balancing Leg Exercise #2	Strength-Building Leg Exercise #2
	Strength-Building Core Exercise #2	Muscle-Balancing Core Exercise #2	Strength-Building Core Exercise #2
	Strength-Building Upper Body Exercise #2	Muscle-Balancing Upper Body Exercise #2	Strength-Building Upper Body Exercise #2
	Strength-Building Leg Exercise #3	Muscle-Balancing Leg Exercise #3	Strength-Building Leg Exercise #3
	Strength-Building Core Exercise #3	Muscle-Balancing Core Exercise #3	Strength-Building Core Exercise #3
	Strength-Building Upper Body Exercise #3	Muscle-Balancing Upper Body Exercise #3	Strength-Building Upper Body Exercise #3
	Strength-Building Leg Exercise #4	Muscle-Balancing Leg Exercise #4	Strength-Building Leg Exercise #4
	Strength-Building Core Exercise #4	Muscle-Balancing Core Exercise #4	Strength-Building Core Exercise #4
	Strength-Building Upper Body Exercise #4	Muscle-Balancing Upper Body Exercise #4	Strength-Building Upper Body Exercise #4

Wk #	Monday	Wednesday	Friday
7	Strength-Building Resistance Workout	Muscle-Balancing Resistance Workout	Strength-Building Resistance Workout
	Summary 3 circuits 12 exercises 39 minutes	Summary 3 circuits 12 exercises 39 minutes	Summary 3 circuits 12 exercises 39 minutes
	Workout:	Workout:	Workout:
	Warm-up	Warm-up	Warm-up
	3X Strength-Building Leg Exercise #1	3X Muscle-Balancing Leg Exercise #1	3X Strength-Building Leg Exercise #1
	Strength-Building Core Exercise #1	Muscle-Balancing Core Exercise #1	Strength-Building Core Exercise #1
	Strength-Building Upper Body Exercise #1	Muscle-Balancing Upper Body Exercise #1	Strength-Building Upper Body Exercise #1
	Strength-Building Leg Exercise #2	Muscle-Balancing Leg Exercise #2	Strength-Building Leg Exercise #2
	Strength-Building Core Fxercise #2	Muscle-Balancing Core Exercise #2	Strength-Building Core Exercise #2
	Strength-Building Upper Body Exercise #2	Muscle-Balancing Upper Body Exercise #2	Strength-Buildıng Upper Body Exercise #2
	Strength-Building Leg Exercise #3	Muscle-Balancing Leg Exercise #3	Strength-Building Leg Exercise #3
	Strength-Building Core Exercise #3	Muscle-Balancing Core Exercise #3	Strength-Building Core Exercise #3
	Strength-Building Upper Body Exercise #3	Muscle-Balancing Upper Body Exercise #3	Strength-Building Upper Body Exercise #3
	Strength-Building Leg Exercise #4	Muscle-Balancing Leg Exercise #4	Strength-Building Leg Exercise #4
	Strength-Building Core Exercise #4	Muscle-Balancing Core Exercise #4	Strength-Building Core Exercise #4
	Strength-Building Upper Body Exercise #4	Muscle-Balancing Upper Body Exercise #4	Strength-Building Upper Body Exercise #4

Wk #	Monday	Wednesday	Friday
8	Strength-Building Resistance Workout	Muscle-Balancing Resistance Workout	Strength-Building Resistance Workout
	Summary 2 circuits 12 exercises 27 minutes	Summary 2 circuits 12 exercises 27 minutes	Summary 2 circuits 12 exercises 27 minutes
	Workout:	Workout:	Workout:
	Warm-up	Warm-up	Warm-up
	2X Strength-Building Leg Exercise #1	2X Muscle-Balancing Leg Exercise #1	2X Strength-Building Leg Exercise #1
	Strength-Building Core Exercise #1	Muscle-Balancing Core Exercise #1	Strength-Building Core Exercise #1
	Strength-Building Upper Body Exercise #1	Muscle-Balancing Upper Body Exercise #1	Strength-Building Upper Body Exercise #1
	Strength-Building Leg Exercise #2	Muscle-Balancing Leg Exercise #2	Strength-Building Leg Exercise #2
	Strength-Building Core Exercise #2	Muscle-Balancing Core Exercise #2	Strength-Building Core Exercise #2
	Strength-Building Upper Body Exercise #2	Muscle-Balancing Upper Body Exercise #2	Strength-Building Upper Body Exercise #2
	Strength-Building Leg Exercise #3	Muscle-Balancing Leg Exercise #3	Strength-Building Leg Exercise #3
	Strength-Building Core Exercise #3	Muscle-Balancing Core Exercise #3	Strength-Building Core Exercise #3
	Strength-Building Upper Body Exercise #3	Muscle-Balancing Upper Body Exercise #3	Strength-Building Upper Body Exercise #3
	Strength-Building Leg Exercise #4	Muscle-Balancing Leg Exercise #4	Strength-Building Leg Exercise #4
	Strength-Building Core Exercise #4	Muscle-Balancing Core Exercise #4	Strength-Building Core Exercise #4
	Strength-Building Upper Body Exercise #4	Muscle-Balancing Upper Body Exercise #4	Strength-Building Upper Body Exercise #4

CHAPTER 11

Cardio Exercise: Intermediate Intervals

I f the cardio training you did in Phase I of the Lean Look program was about getting off to a fast start, the cardio training in Phase II is about building momentum. The differences are subtle yet sufficient to take your progress to the next level. Throughout Phase II you will perform two intermediate interval cardio workouts per week: 2-minute intervals on Thursday and 3-minute intervals on Saturday. Somewhat more challenging than your short interval workouts, these intermediate interval workouts will burn even more fat and boost your aerobic fitness. On Tuesday you will continue doing the 1-minute intervals you did in Phase I. Speed and power intervals are phased out in Phase II.

You will start with a challenging but manageable version of

each new cardio workout in Week 5, then move to longer interval workouts consisting of more intervals in subsequent weeks before returning to the Week 5 workout in Week 8, which is a recovery week. As you will see in consulting the cardio exercise schedules later in this chapter, the shortest 2-minute interval workout occurs in Week 8 of the beginner schedule; it includes four total intervals and takes 24 minutes to complete. The longest two-minute interval workout includes six total intervals and takes 32 minutes to complete; it is done in weeks 6 and 7 of the advanced schedule. The shortest 3-minute interval workout is found in Week 5 of the beginner schedule; it includes three intervals and is 25 minutes long. The longest 3-minute interval workout falls in Week 7 of the advanced schedule; it features five intervals and lasts 37 minutes.

Use the plus-one rule to guide your level of effort in your 2-minute and 3-minute interval workouts. In these workouts you should complete the last interval at the same pace at which you started the first interval and feel as though you could do one and only one more interval at the same pace if you had to. Naturally, because they are shorter, you will be able to work a little harder in your 2-minute intervals than in your 3-minute intervals, but you won't be able to work as intensely in either your 2- or 3-minute intervals as you did in the three shorter types of interval workouts introduced in Phase I. As with the short intervals you did in Phase I, you might have to fiddle around with different combinations of pace and resistance before you find the level of effort that's best for your intermediate intervals.

Begin your intermediate interval workouts with a 5-minute warm-up at a moderate level of effort in your chosen cardio activity. Again, it's very important that you complete a gentle, thorough warm-up to warm, lubricate, and oxygenate your muscles, preparing them to work harder effectively and without undue strain. When starting the first higher-intensity interval, increase the effort level from your warm-up effort by increasing your pace, your resistance level, or both, as appropriate. After completing each higher-intensity interval, do a moderate-intensity active recovery that's equal in duration to the higher-intensity interval you just completed, except after the last interval, when you should proceed straight to a 5-minute cooldown. Here's a more detailed look at the structure of the 2-minute and 3-minute interval cardio workouts.

2-MINUTE INTERVALS

Warm up with 5 minutes of moderate-intensity movement in your chosen activity. Next increase your level of effort by increasing your pace and/or resistance for 2 minutes. Use the plus-one rule to guide your effort. After completing the 2-minute interval, slow back down to your warm-up effort level for 2 minutes of active recovery. Once you've completed the prescribed number of 2-minute higher-intensity intervals, cool down for 5 minutes. Do not perform a 2-minute active recovery following your last 2-minute interval, but instead go straight to the 5-minute cooldown. Thus a 2-minute intervals workout featuring 4 intervals looks like this:

5-minute easy warm-up

2 minutes hard

2-minute active recovery

2 minutes hard

2-minute active recovery

2 minutes hard

2-minute active recovery

2 minutes hard

5-minute easy cooldown

Total time: 24 minutes

3-MINUTE INTERVALS

Warm up with 5 minutes of moderate-intensity movement in your chosen activity. Next increase your level of effort by increasing your pace and/or resistance for 3 minutes. Use the plus-one rule to guide your effort. After completing the 3-minute interval, slow back down to your warm-up effort level for 3 minutes of active recovery. Once you've completed the prescribed number of 3-minute higher-intensity intervals, cool down for 5 minutes. Do not perform a 3-minute active recovery following your last 3-minute interval, but instead go straight to the 5-minute cooldown. Thus a 3-minute intervals workout featuring 4 intervals looks like this:

5-minute easy warm-up

3 minutes hard

3-minute active recovery

3 minutes hard

3-minute active recovery

3 minutes hard

3-minute active recovery

3 minutes hard

5-minute easy cooldown

Total time: 31 minutes

Continue to adapt your cardio workouts to whichever form or forms of cardio exercise you prefer. The following charts provide detailed Phase II cardio workout schedules for the beginner and advanced levels. Intervals of all three types included in this phase—2-minute, 1-minute, and 3-minute intervals—are designated by the word "hard," but remember that the precise level of effort should be slightly different in each type of workout.

SQUASHING THE INJURY BUG

I would like to devote the remainder of this chapter to the subject of preventing overuse injuries. Overuse injuries such as tendonitis are all too common among those who participate in repetitive cardio activities, including swimming, cycling, and running, and these injuries are particularly common among relative beginners. As you ramp up your cardio training in Phase II of the Lean Look program, you will want to do everything possible to minimize the risk of having your progress derailed by a sore knee, shin splints, or the like.

As the name suggests, overuse injuries are caused by overusing certain parts of the body. You can repeat a specific motion only so many times before some of the tissues involved begin to wear down. Overuse injuries involve the

PHASE II CARDIO EXERCISE—BEGINNER SCHEDULE

5	2-Minute Intervals	1-Minute Intervals	3-Minute Intervals
	5-minute easy warm-up 4 X (2 minutes hard/ 2 minutes easy) 5-minute easy cooldown	5-minute easy warm-up 6 X (1 minute hard/ 1 minute easy) 5-minute easy cooldown	5-minute easy warm-up 3 X (3 minutes hard/ 3 minutes easy) 5-minute easy cooldown
	Total time: 24 minutes	Total time: 21 minutes	Total time: 25 minutes
6	2-Minute Intervals	1-Minute Intervals	3-Minute Intervals
	5-minute easy warm-up 5 X (2 minutes hard/ 2 minutes easy) 5-minute easy cooldown	5-minute easy warm-up 7 X (1 minute hard/ 1 minute easy) 5-minute easy cooldown	5-minute easy warm-up 3 X (3 minutes hard/ 3 minutes easy) 5-minute easy cooldown
	Total time: 28 minutes	Total time: 23 minutes	Total time: 25 minutes
7	2-Minute Intervals	1-Minute Intervals	3-Minute Intervals
	5-minute easy warm-up 5 X (2 minutes hard/ 2 minutes easy) 5-minute easy cooldown	5-minute easy warm-up 8 X (1 minute hard/ 1 minute easy) 5-minute easy cooldown	5-minute easy warm-up 4 X (3 minutes hard/ 3 minutes easy) 5-minute easy cooldown
	Total time: 28 minutes	Total time: 25 minutes	Total time: 31 minutes
8	2-Minute Intervals	1-Minute Intervals	3-Minute Intervals
	5-minute easy warm-up 4 X (2 minutes hard/ 2 minutes easy) 5-minute easy cooldown	5-minute easy warm-up 6 X (1 minute hard/ 1 minute easy) 5-minute easy cooldown	5-minute easy warm-up 3 X (3 minutes hard/ 3 minutes easy) 5-minute easy cooldown
	Total time: 24 minutes	Total time: 21 minutes	Total time: 25 minutes

PHASE II

gradual breakdown of body tissues resulting from repetitive motion over the course of days, weeks, or even months. As such, these injuries are quite different from so-called acute injuries, including ankle sprains. Most overuse injuries are preventable. While doing too much will always result in a breakdown eventually, taking certain precautions will increase the amount of activity you can do without developing an injury.

Effective injury-prevention measures include warming up properly, maintaining correct form in your cardio activities, wearing properly fitting athletic

PHASE II CARDIO EXERCISE—ADVANCED SCHEDULE

Wk #	Tuesday	Thursday	Saturday
5	2-Minute Intervals 5-minute easy warm-up 5 X (2 minutes hard/ 2 minutes easy) 5-minute easy cooldown Total time: 28 minutes	1-Minute Intervals 5-minute easy warm-up 8 X (1 minute hard/ 1 minute easy) 5-minute easy cooldown Total time: 25 minutes	3-Minute Intervals 5-minute easy warm-up 4 X (3 minutes hard/ 3 minutes easy) 5-minute easy cooldown Total time: 31 minutes
6	2-Minute Intervals 5-minute easy warm-up 6 X (2 minutes hard/ 2 minutes easy) 5-minute easy cooldown Total time: 32 minutes	1-Minute Intervals 5-minute easy warm-up 9 X (1 minute hard/ 1 minute easy) 5-minute easy cooldown Total time: 27 minutes	3-Minute Intervals 5-minute easy warm-up 4 X (3 minutes hard/ 3 minutes easy) 5-minute easy cooldown Total time: 31 minutes
7	2-Minute Intervals 5-minute easy warm-up 6 X (2 minutes hard/ 2 minutes easy) 5-minute easy cooldown Total time: 32 minutes	1-Minute Intervals 5-minute easy warm-up 10 X (1 minute hard/ 1 minute easy) 5-minute easy cooldown Total time: 29 minutes	3-Minute Intervals 5-minute easy warm-up 5 X (3 minutes hard/ 3 minutes easy) 5-minute easy cooldown Total time: 37 minutes
8	2-Minute Intervals 5-minute easy warm-up 5 X (2 minutes hard/ 2 minutes easy) 5-minute easy cooldown Total time: 28 minutes	1-Minute Intervals 5-minute easy warm-up 8 X (1 minute hard/ 1 minute easy) 5-minute easy cooldown Total time: 25 minutes	3-Minute Intervals 5-minute easy warm-up 4 X (3 minutes hard/ 3 minutes easy) 5-minute easy cooldown Total time: 31 minutes

shoes and replacing them before they get too worn, and varying your workouts—for example, swimming one day, running one day, and bicycling one day a week instead of swimming, cycling, or running three times a week. Varying your activity limits the amount of repetition you experience in any single movement.

Many overuse injuries are caused by muscle imbalances; that is, by weakness in certain important stabilizing muscles (muscles that keep the joints stable during an activity) or by excessive tightness in muscles (or tendons). For example, in runners, weak hip abductors (the muscles on the outside of the hip) can cause the pelvis to tip toward your unsupported side when your foot lands, placing undue strain on the hip and/or knee joints. Many cycling injuries are associated with muscle imbalances that develop as a result of spending a lot of time maintaining a hunched cycling posture while pedaling. Lower back pain is an especially common complaint among those who do their cardio exercise on a bike. The muscle imbalances associated with swimmer's shoulder (a form of bursitis) are tightness in the chest, medial shoulder rotators, and lower back, and weakness in the rotator cuff muscles, the scapular stabilizers, and the lower abdomen.

The resistance-training component of the Lean Look program will improve your muscle balance by strengthening joint-stabilizing muscles throughout your body, and thereby prevent some overuse injuries. But in order to improve your muscle balance further, you also need to stretch certain muscles and tendons that tend to cause overuse injuries when they are too tight.

Do the following stretches at least three times a week at any time of day except first thing in the morning, when the spine in particular is less flexible. Stretch any "problem" muscles and tendons daily.

Chest Stretch

Lift your arms straight to the sides, palms forward, and press them backward until you feel a stretch in your chest muscles. Hold this position for 15 seconds.

Biceps and Front Shoulder Stretch

Stand with your arms at your sides and your palms turned inward. Raise your arms behind your body until you feel a stretch in the front of your shoulders and in your biceps. Hold this position for 15 seconds.

Rotator Cuff Stretches

To stretch your internal shoulder rotators, raise your arms in a "Don't shoot" position and press your elbows backward until you feel a stretch in your shoulders. Hold this position for 15 seconds.

To stretch your external shoulder rotators, from the "Don't shoot" position, rotate your shoulders forward 180 degrees so that your fingers are now pointing toward the floor and your palms are facing backward. Again, press your elbows backward until you feel a stretch in your shoulders. Hold this position for 15 seconds.

Back Stretch

Reach your arms straight overhead and lace your fingers together. Lean to the left until you feel a stretch in the right side of your back. Hold this position for 15 seconds and then lean to the right.

Hip Flexors Stretch

Kneel on your left knee and place your right foot on the floor well in front of your body. Draw your navel toward your spine and roll your pelvis backward. Now put your weight forward into the lunge until you feel a good stretch in your left hip flexors (located where your thigh joins your pelvis). You can extend the stretch to your psoas (a pair of hip flexor muscles connecting your pelvis and spine) by raising your left arm over your head and actively reaching toward the ceiling. Hold the stretch for 20 seconds and then repeat on the right side.

Quadriceps Stretch

Stand on your left foot, bend your right leg fully, and grab your right foot with your right hand behind you. Gently pull on your foot until you feel a stretch in the front of your right thigh. Hold the stretch for 20 seconds and then repeat on the left side.

Hamstrings Stretch

Lay on your back with both legs bent. Begin with one foot resting flat on the floor and the other leg elevated so that the thigh is perpendicular to the floor and the shin is parallel to the floor. Loop a strap or rope around the bottom of this foot and grasp the two segments together next to your knee using the hand on the same side of your body as the leg that is being stretched. By contracting your quadriceps, straighten the rope-looped leg completely. Gently tug on the ends of the rope until you feel a good stretch in your hamstrings. Hold it for 1 to 2 seconds and relax. Repeat this stretch a total of 10 times, then stretch the opposite leg.

Groin Stretch

Sit on the floor with your legs sharply bent and the bottoms of your feet together. Grasp your feet with your hands and gently pull your torso forward until you feel a stretch in your inner thighs. Hold the stretch for 20 seconds.

Iliotibial Band Stretch

Stand with your legs crossed so that your left foot is planted several inches to the right of your right foot. Sink your weight into your right hip socket and tip your torso to the left (but remain facing forward). You should begin to feel a stretch at the top of your iliotibial (IT) band, just beneath your hip bone. Hold this stretch for 20 seconds and then cross your right leg over your left to stretch the left IT band.

Buttocks Stretch

Stand on your left foot, bend your left leg slightly, and cross your right leg over the left so that the outside of your lower right shin is resting against your lower left thigh. Use your hands to hold your right leg in this position. Now sink your butt a few inches toward the floor and use your hands to rotate your right leg outward until you feel a stretch in your right buttock. Hold this stretch for 15 seconds and then reverse your position and stretch the left side.

Calf Stretch

Stand on the edge of a step. Place the ball of your left foot at the very edge so that your heel is unsupported. Drop your left heel toward the floor while keeping your leg straight. Hold this stretch for 20 seconds. This will stretch the gastrocnemius, which is the larger, more visible muscle in your calf. Now bend your knee slightly and feel the stretch migrate downward into your soleus muscle. Hold this stretch for 20 seconds. Now stretch the right side.

Achilles Tendon Stretch

Stand in a split stance, one foot a step ahead of the other, with both feet flat on the ground and both knees slightly bent. Now bend your back leg a little more and concentrate on trying to "sink" your butt straight down toward the heel of that foot. Keep your torso upright. You should begin to feel a stretch in your Achilles tendon. You may have to fiddle with your position before you find that stretch. Now stretch the opposite leg. When you do, hold it for 10 or 12 seconds, relax, and then stretch it a couple more times.

PHASE III

CHAPTER 12

Introduction
to Phase III

In Phase III of the Lean Look program you will have the option of adding nutritional supplements to your diet while still practicing the ten key food substitutions you took up in Phase I and the eight nutrient timing habits you learned in Phase II. You will also continue to perform three resistance workouts and three cardio workouts per week, but the nature of these workouts will change.

The focus of your resistance workouts will shift from strength building to power development. On the cardio side, you will transition to a schedule of two long interval workouts and one intermediate-length interval workout per week. Finally, don't forget to measure your body fat percentage once a week throughout Phase III, as you did in the first eight weeks of the program.

NUTRITION: SMART SUPPLEMENTATION

Many Americans are skeptical of the practice of nutritional supplementation because the supplements industry is not well regulated, and as a result misleading marketing practices are rampant and products lacking any scientific evidence of their benefits are legion. Nevertheless, there are a small handful of nutritional supplements that are scientifically proven to enhance leanness and overall health.

Supplementation is never necessary to achieve the Lean Look or optimal health, and this practice should never be relied on too heavily. I don't pressure my clients to use supplements and I want it to be clear that nutritional supplementation is 100 percent optional. Indeed, the reason I have delayed the introduction of supplementation until Phase III is that I want to emphasize the greater importance of key food substitutions and nutrient timing in relation to the Lean Look and optimal health.

There are seven nutritional supplements that I believe to be worth considering, based on solid scientific evidence supporting their benefits, and I'll introduce them in the next chapter.

RESISTANCE EXERCISE: POWER DEVELOPMENT

In Phase I you created a solid foundation for muscle building and started the process of increasing the size and strength of your muscles. In Phase II you built strength on top of the foundation laid in Phase I. Now, in Phase III, you will shift to doing one power-developing resistance workout and two strength-building resistance workouts per week. The addition of power-developing resistance workouts to your routine, in combination with doing longer strength-building resistance workouts, will enable you to achieve peak muscular fitness by requiring your muscles to adapt to a new challenge. In Chapter 14 I will introduce you to a whole new pool of resistance exercises that are great for building power.

CARDIO EXERCISE: LONG INTERVALS

The cardio training emphasis of Phase III is long intervals of 4 to 6 minutes. Long intervals are very challenging because they are performed at a relatively high intensity despite their extended duration. To get the most out of long intervals, you need to have established a solid foundation of cardio fitness. That's why long intervals are introduced in Phase III instead of earlier. The payoff you get from taking on the challenge of long intervals is that you will get even leaner and elevate your cardiovascular fitness to even greater heights.

In Phase III you will begin doing cardio workouts featuring 6-minute intervals on Tuesdays and cardio workouts featuring 4-minute intervals on Saturdays. On Thursdays you will do cardio workouts featuring intermediate intervals of either 2 or 3 minutes. Chapter 15 provides detailed guidelines for these new cardio workouts.

WORKOUT SCHEDULES

On the following pages are general resistance and cardio workout schedules for Phase III of the Lean Look program. Chapters 14 and 15 provide more detailed information about how to do your Phase III resistance workouts and cardio workouts. After you have read through all of the text on Phase III, refer back to the charts provided here, which show you how your resistance workouts and cardio workouts fit together week by week.

BEGINNER SCHEDULE

The chart on the next page lists the general Phase III resistance and cardio workout schedule for the beginner exercise level. Use this workout schedule if you started with the beginner schedule in Phase I, or if you started with the advanced schedule in Phase I but are finding the workouts too challenging or are having trouble recovering fully between workouts.

PHASE III

199

Wk #	Monday	Tuesday	Wednesday	Thursday	Friday	Saturday
9	Resistance (Strength-Building) 3 circuits 9 exercises 30 minutes	Cardio (6-minute intervals) 2 intervals 25 minutes	Resistance (Power Development) 2 circuits 9 exercises 21 minutes	Cardio (2-minute intervals) 3 intervals 20 minutes	Resistance (Strength-Building) 2 circuits 9 exercises 21 minutes	Cardio (4-minute intervals) 2 intervals 20 minutes
10	Resistance (Strength-Building) 3 circuits 9 exercises 30 minutes	Cardio (6-minute intervals) 2 intervals 25 minutes	Resistance (Power Development) 3 circuits 9 exercises 30 minutes	Cardio (3-minute intervals) 3 intervals 25 minutes	Resistance (Strength-Building) 3 circuits 9 exercises 30 minutes	Cardio (4-minute intervals) 3 intervals 26 minutes
11	Resistance (Strength-Building) 3 circuits 9 exercises 30 minutes	Cardio (6-minute intervals) 3 intervals 34 minutes	Resistance (Power Development) 3 circuits 9 exercises 30 minutes	Cardio (2-minute intervals) 4 intervals 24 minutes	Resistance (Strength-Building) 3 circuits 9 exercises 30 minutes	Cardio (4-minute intervals) 3 intervals 26 minutes
12	Resistance (Strength-Building) 3 circuits 9 exercises 21 minutes	Cardio (6-minute intervals) 2 intervals 25 minutes	Resistance (Power Development) 2 circuits 9 exercises 21 minutes	Cardio (3-minute intervals) 3 intervals 25 minutes	Resistance (Strength-Building) 2 circuits 9 exercises 21 minutes	Cardio (4-minute intervals) 2 intervals 20 minutes

ADVANCED SCHEDULE

Use this workout schedule if you started with the advanced schedule in Phase I and have not found the workouts in this schedule too challenging.

Wk #	Monday	Tuesday	Wednesday	Thursday	Friday	Saturday
9	Resistance (Strength-Building)	Cardio (6-minute intervals)	Resistance (Power Development)	Cardio (2-minute intervals)	Resistance (Strength-Building)	Cardio (4-minute intervals)
	3 circuits 12 exercises	3 intervals	2 circuits 12 exercises	4 intervals	3 circuits 12 exercises	3 intervals
	39 minutes	34 minutes	27 minutes	24 minutes	39 minutes	26 minutes
10	Resistance (Strength-Building)	Cardio (6-minute intervals)	Resistance (Power Development)	Cardio (3-minute intervals)	Resistance (Strength-Building)	Cardio (4-minute intervals)
	3 circuits 12 exercises	3 intervals	3 circuits 12 exercises	4 intervals	3 circuits 12 exercises	4 intervals
	39 minutes	34 minutes	39 minutes	31 minutes	39 minutes	32 minutes
11	Resistance (Strength-Building)	Cardio (6-minute intervals)	Resistance (Power Development)	Cardio (2-minute intervals)	Resistance (Strength-Building)	Cardio (4-minute intervals)
	3 circuits 12 exercises	4 intervals	3 circuits 12 exercises	5 intervals	3 circuits 12 exercises	4 intervals
	39 minutes	43 minutes	39 minutes	28 minutes	39 minutes	32 minutes
12	Resistance (Strength-Building)	Cardio (6-minute intervals)	Resistance (Power Development)	Cardio (3-minute intervals)	Resistance (Strength-Building)	Cardio (4-minute intervals)
	2 circuits 12 exercises	3 intervals	2 circuits 12 exercises	4 intervals	2 circuits 12 exercises	3 intervals
	27 minutes	34 minutes	27 minutes	31 minutes	27 minutes	26 minutes

CHAPTER 13

Nutrition: Smart Supplementation

Nutritional supplements are a controversial topic these days. At one extreme of the debate are natural food advocates who argue that nutritional supplements are at best a useless waste of money and in the worst cases actually *harmful* to human health. They claim that our bodies are designed to make use of only the organic, unprocessed foods that our earliest ancestors survived on many thousands of years ago. To consume unnaturally large doses of individual nutrients extracted from natural foods (which is the essence of supplementation) is, they insist, to risk throwing our bodies off balance in one way or another, and therefore it shouldn't be done. At the other extreme of the debate is the multibillion-dollar supplements industry, which has a bottom-line interest in convincing consumers that specific supplements are beneficial, if not necessary, for optimal health, and the medical science–marketing machine that gives credibility to at least some of the claims of the supplement companies.

The truth, as usual, lies midway between these extremes. Those who categorically dismiss all supplements as useless or harmful are allowing ideology to cloud their vision. On the other hand, supplement makers and those "experts" with ties to them frequently put self-interest ahead of honesty. A clear-eyed, case-by-case look at the scientific information concerning each supplement leads to a more moderate conclusion. The reality is that most nutritional supplements are useless, and, yes, a few are potentially harmful when consumed in excess. But some nutritional supplements offer benefits that natural foods can't match, or they provide the same benefits as natural foods in a more convenient way.

Let me be clear: Without question, the overwhelming majority of your daily nutrition should come from natural foods such as fish and fresh vegetables. However there are a very few key nutritional supplements that you can layer on top of a solid foundation of natural foods to take your quest for the Lean Look even further. In this chapter I would like to introduce you to this small handful of supplements and give you the option of incorporating them into Phase III of the Lean Look program. I have deliberately chosen to save the introduction of nutritional supplements until Phase III and to present supplementation as optional because I wish to send a plain message that getting your everyday diet right is a higher priority. Too many men and women approach supplements with a magic bullet mentality, hoping that a handful of pills can take the place of a proper diet or make up for bad eating habits. They can't. There are no "miracle" nutritional supplements. Nor are there any supplements that can be considered truly necessary for optimal body composition and health. You can still achieve your optimal body composition and health without taking any supplements. In fact, plenty of my clients choose not to rely on any supplements.

A typical example is John, a forty-one-year-old husband, father, and busy career man who came to me with a goal of dropping from his current weight of 183 pounds back down to his college weight of 170 pounds. We translated this goal into body fat percentage terms and then promptly achieved it by making three simple changes to his diet. I asked John to eat a heartier, healthier breakfast each morning, to pack his own lunch and take it to work, and to eat two or three healthy snacks throughout the day. That's it! No supplements necessary.

Nevertheless, making judicious use of appropriate supplements is a safe and effective way to fine-tune your nutrition in Phase III of the Lean Look program (and beyond), after you have established a solid foundation with the key substitutions of Phase I and the nutrient timing practices of Phase II.

Here's how I recommend you approach the nutrition component of Phase III of the Lean Look program. First, read through this chapter and note the benefits and usage recommendations for each supplement discussed. Next, use this information to decide which of these supplements you wish to try, if any. Finally, begin using your chosen supplements according to label directions on a trial basis, and see how they work for you. If you like what they do for you, keep using them. If you decide they aren't worth the money, stop using them. It's as simple as that.

SEVEN SUPPLEMENTS TO CONSIDER

The following seven supplements represent three basic categories: those that promote leanness by enhancing workout performance and recovery; those that promote leanness by reducing fat storage; and those that promote general health and, in so doing, may indirectly promote leanness—with some overlap among categories.

BETA-ALANINE

Beta-alanine is a nonessential amino acid that is obtained in the diet primarily from meats containing carnosine, a naturally occurring peptide made up of beta-alanine and L-histidine. Beta-alanine serves a variety of functions in the body, but perhaps its most important role is to help formulate carnosine, which is not absorbed intact from food sources.

Carnosine has long been celebrated as an "antiaging" compound because it is an antioxidant, prevents glycation (a process whereby excess sugar in the bloodstream damages body proteins, contributing to Alzheimer's disease and

BETA-ALANINE SUPPLEMENTS

Beta-X High Performance Beta-Alanine

Body Octane (MAN Sports)

H+Blocker (iSatori Technologies)

IntraXCell Intracellular Carnosine Booster

Muscle-Link Red Dragon

other problems), and extends the life span of individual cells. But more recently scientists have discovered that carnosine has a powerful role in exercise performance. Specifically, it helps the muscles maintain normal pH levels during intense exercise, when there is a tendency for the muscles to become too acidic, causing fatigue (and that burning sensation you may be familiar with).

Consistent, high-intensity exercise naturally increases the muscle carnosine concentration, but research has shown that taking a daily beta-alanine supplement increases it far more than training and a carnosine-rich diet can. As muscle carnosine levels increase, performance in high-intensity workouts (such as the resistance and cardio workouts you're doing in the Lean Look program) improves. For example, a joint study by British and South Korean researchers found that four weeks of supplementation with beta-alanine increased the muscle concentration of carnosine by 64 percent and increased anaerobic exercise performance by 14 percent. By increasing your muscle carnosine stores through beta-alanine supplementation, you will be able to maintain a higher work level in both your muscle toning workouts and your cardio workouts, and as a result you will build muscle and shed fat faster.

There are several beta-alanine supplements on the market that are formulated especially for exercisers, and I've listed them in the box above. Some also contain L-histidine or other nutrients. The beta-alanine dosage level that has been proven effective in studies is 3–6 grams daily; I would say 1–4 grams daily is plenty.

I should note that there is one strange but totally harmless side effect of beta-alanine supplementation, which affects roughly half of those who take it. Parathesia is a fancy name for a transient and benign tingling sensation in the upper extremities resulting from beta-alanine's actions as a neurotransmitter. High levels of beta-alanine supplementation have also been known to result in taurine depletion (i.e., reduced cellular stores of the amino acid taurine), which may make concomitant taurine supplementation advisable.

CREATINE

Creatine phosphate occurs naturally in the body and is one of the most important sources of energy for high-intensity (anaerobic) muscle contractions. Creatine phosphate can provide energy so rapidly that it is the muscles' primary energy source for maximum-intensity efforts such as heavy weight lifting and sprinting. The muscles store it in extremely small amounts, though, so it lasts no longer than 15 seconds during maximum-intensity muscle work.

A tiny percentage of our creatine phosphate stores is synthesized in the body. The rest comes ready-made in protein-rich foods, including fish and beef. But even these foods contain only very small amounts of creatine phosphate. That's why scientists in the 1990s began to look at creatine supplementation as a potential means to enhance high-intensity muscle performance (strength, speed, and power) by increasing the availability of this particular energy source in the muscles. They quickly found that various creatine phosphate precursors, including creatine monohydrate, are readily converted to creatine phosphate in the body and, when taken supplementally, increase creatine phosphate stores in the muscles far beyond the levels that can be achieved by diet alone.

CREATINE SUPPLEMENTS

EAS Phosphagen Elite
GNC Pro Performance® Creatine Monohydrate
Meta-Cel (iSatori Technologies)
MuscleTech® Creakic
TwinLab Creatine Fuel

As few as five days of creatine monohydrate supplementation increase creatine phosphate levels in the body by 10 to 40 percent. Dozens of research studies have shown that these increases translate directly into faster muscle development and strength building. Don't worry—creatine supplements are not anything like anabolic steroids; they don't increase muscle size or strength nearly as much as steroids do, and they have no side effects. But I have known a few individuals who have found them to be too effective for their liking. If you tend to gain muscle mass very easily and are not interested in becoming extremely muscular, creatine supplements might not be for you. Others find creatine to have little effect. Scientists refer to these individuals as "non-responders." Even among the majority of men and women who do respond to creatine supplementation, some benefit more than others, so if you're interested in trying creatine, you'll just have to see how it works for you.

I recommend that you take 2 to 3 grams per day (not the 5 grams per day that most labels indicate). Because insulin is needed to drive creatine into the muscle cells, you should mix the powder into fruit juice (or take the pills with fruit juice). Otherwise you can buy the supplement as a flavored drink mix.

There has been some public concern about side effects associated with creatine supplementation, including muscle cramping and altered liver and kidney function. However, formal scientific studies have found no evidence of any side effects, except muscle weight gain, and recent comprehensive reviews of the literature have concluded that even long-term creatine supplementation is safe.

Most long-term creatine users take creatine in cycles (normally 8–12 weeks on, 2–4 weeks off), which is done mainly to avoid building too great a "tolerance" for ingested creatine rather than for health reasons.

FIBER

Fiber (also known as roughage) is the name given to two kinds of highly complex carbohydrates that are totally indigestible. Although fiber is technically a carbohydrate, unlike other forms of carbohydrate (sugars and starches), it provides no calories because it is not absorbed into the bloodstream. Insoluble fiber (mainly cellulose) serves as an important structural material in plants. It does not provide nutrition to humans but benefits us instead by ab-

---

FIBER SUPPLEMENTS

Benefiber	Citrucel
FiberCon	Metamucil

---

sorbing and neutralizing toxins and by contributing to well-hydrated, bulky solid waste that is easily passed. Water-soluble fiber helps the body absorb minerals and helps remove nutrient excesses, including cholesterol, from the body. Examples of fiber-rich foods are whole grains, green leafy vegetables, and beans.

Adequate fiber intake is essential for optimal health; conversely, inadequate fiber intake is associated with a variety of diseases and health conditions. Specifically, a high-fiber diet is known to reduce the risk of obesity, type 2 diabetes, cardiovascular disease, and constipation. One of the reasons these diseases and conditions are so prevalent in our society is that we do not consume enough dietary fiber. The U.S. Surgeon General and many professional health organizations recommend a diet containing 20–35 grams of fiber a day. The average American consumes a scant 10–15 grams daily.

Excess body fat is the primary cause of cardiovascular disease and type 2 diabetes. A high-fiber diet may reduce the risk of cardiovascular disease and type 2 diabetes by reducing the storage of body fat. Fiber slows digestion so we feel fuller longer and consequently eat less. Therefore getting enough fiber in your diet is very beneficial when it comes to achieving the Lean Look. A few of the key dietary substitutions I recommended in chapter 5 are essentially ways of getting more fiber in your diet.

Natural foods such as fruits and vegetables are the best sources of dietary fiber, but fiber supplements can be a good backup source. If you are currently getting less than 35 grams of fiber daily and you're finding it difficult to add more whole grains, fruits, or vegetables to your diet, use a supplement such as ground flax seeds or one of those fiber supplements listed above. Use it according to label directions and aim for a total of roughly 35 grams of fiber daily from food and supplement sources combined.

FISH OIL/FLAXSEED OIL

Omega-3 fatty acids are a type of essential fatty acid (EFA) that cannot be synthesized in the body and must be obtained in adequate amounts in the diet. This is easier said than done, because omega-3 fatty acids are destroyed when the oils that contain them are processed or heated, and most of the omega-3 sources in the modern diet are processed and/or heated. Many experts believe that omega-3 deficiency is one of the most widespread nutrient deficiencies in our society. It is certainly the most common nutrient deficiency in my clients' diets.

Omega-3 EFAs create healthier cell membranes. In addition, they are important precursors to anti-inflammatory components of the immune system. Omega-3 supplementation has been shown to improve cardiovascular health, sympathetic nervous system function, immune function, and skin health. For this reason, and because it is very difficult to get enough omega-3 EFAs from regular foods, omega-3 supplementation is advisable for most people.

The American Heart Association recommends a daily omega-3 intake of 1,000 mg. Intake levels above 3,000 mg per day may be unhealthy. Most omega-3 supplements are formulated to provide 500 to 1,000 mg per serving. Avoid oil supplements that contain omega-3 and omega-6 fatty acids in a ratio of less than 2:1, as omega-6 fatty acids are much easier to come by in the diet and research has shown that the benefits of getting more omega-3s are nullified when you increase your omega-6 intake disproportionately. The most popular EFA supplements are fish oil and flaxseed oil.

FLAXSEED OILS	**FISH OILS**
Puritan's Flax Seed Oil (capsules)	Coromega Omega-3 Fatty Acids
Natural Brand Flax Seed Oil (liquid)	Country Life Omega-3 Fish Oil
Solaray Flaxseed Oil (capsules)	Puritan's Pride Omega-3 EPA Fish Oil

GLUCOSAMINE AND CHONDROITIN

Glucosamine and chondroitin are natural compounds found in joint carti-lage. They have become popular as dietary supplements (usually in the form of glucosamine hydrochloride and chondroitin sulfate) among arthritis suf-ferers, athletes, and others experiencing joint pain and dysfunction.

Recent studies have shown that, both individually and in combination, glucosamine and chondroitin supplements are effective in reducing joint pain associated with damaged cartilage, improving mobility in the affected joint, and limiting further cartilage deterioration. Almost all of these studies have involved patients with osteoarthritis, not runners or other athletes with joint pain caused by activity. Nevertheless, thousands of athletes (especially run-ners) currently take these supplements to protect their joint cartilage from breakdown that could lead to osteoarthritis.

Are glucosamine and chondroitin supplements effective in preventing or treating knee pain and dysfunction in athletes and exercisers? The short an-swer is that no one knows, because this question has not yet been formally studied. However, there is plenty of anecdotal evidence of a positive effect, and most experts speculate that ultimately these supplements will be shown to be beneficial.

There are no official recommended dosages of glucosamine and chon-droitin. The average dosages used in studies that have found a positive effect and no significant side effects are 1500 milligrams per day of glucosamine and 800 milligrams per day of chondroitin. There is believed to be a wide dispar-

---

GLUCOSAMINE AND CHONDROITIN SUPPLEMENTS

GNC Glucosamine 750 Chondroitin 600

Preventive Nutrition Glucosamine Chondroitin

Puritan's Pride Triple Strength Glucosamine Chondroitin

Vitamin World Double Strength Glucosamine Chondroitin

Flex-a-min

ity in the quality (i.e., purity) of various brands, so ask your naturopath or supplements salesperson for recommendations before you buy.

VITAMIN AND MINERAL SUPPLEMENTS

Taking supplemental vitamins and minerals won't make you leaner—at least not directly. But it might make you healthier in other ways, for example by strengthening your immune system. And anything you do that makes you healthier may ultimately have a positive effect on your body composition. For example, the recommended daily intake of calcium is 1,000 to 1,300 milligrams; the average adult consumes only 500 to 700 milligrams daily. The major consequence of this common deficiency is weakening of the bones, which increases the risk of stress fractures in runners and other athletes. But research has also shown that calcium plays an important role in fat metabolism, and when a slight calorie deficit is combined with calcium supplementation, fat burning is increased.

If your diet is rich in fruits and vegetables and quality animal foods, chances are you are already getting optimal amounts of all the essential vitamins and minerals. Taking a quality vitamin and mineral supplement as an adjunct to a healthy diet will remove any last bit of doubt on this matter and will make up for occasional deficiencies in this or that vitamin or mineral on those days when your eating is a little off balance. If your diet is poor, you may need a vitamin or mineral supplement just to prevent health problems related to vitamin and mineral deficiencies. For example, failure to consume adequate

---

VITAMIN AND MINERAL SUPPLEMENTS

All One Green Phyto Base (All One/NutriTech)

Greens Plus

Juice Plus +

Nature's Way Alive! Whole Food Energizer Veggie Capsules

Source of Life (Nature's Plus)

amounts of B vitamins, a common problem these days, results in elevated levels of the amino acid homocysteine in the blood, which is a risk factor for coronary heart disease. But no amount of vitamin and mineral supplementation can completely make up for everything you're missing if you don't consume enough fruits and vegetables. As I tell my clients all the time, "If you supplement a bad diet, you're just supplementing a bad diet."

The most practical and economical way to get all your supplemental vitamins and minerals is from a single supplement source instead of trying to get them from many separate supplements and pills. Don't bother with vitamin and mineral supplements labeled as being especially for women, men, older people, children, or whatever—these are marketing gimmicks. We're all human and we all need the same vitamins and minerals.

It's important to choose a supplement containing nutrients in forms that are well absorbed. Most vitamin and mineral supplements contain vitamins and minerals in forms that are poorly absorbed, meaning the nutrients literally pass straight through your body without ever being metabolized. While no supplement can match the absorption rate of natural foods, "real food" supplements come the closest because they contain extracts from real foods and/or vitamins and minerals in the forms found in real foods. The box on page 211 provides examples of "real food" vitamin and mineral supplements.

When choosing and using vitamin and mineral supplements, it's important to keep the following recommendations in mind:

• Look for supplements that contain at least 50 percent of the USRDA of each vitamin and mineral ingredient.

• Avoid supplements that contain more than 200 percent of the USRDA of individual vitamins and minerals. There is such a thing as too much.

• In traditional vitamin and mineral supplements (i.e., pills containing stripped-down, individual vitamins and minerals), look for the letters "USP" on the supplement bottle. This stands for "United States Pharmacopoeia." Only vitamin and mineral supplements of the highest quality and absorbability earn this designation.

• Alternatively, look for the "CL Approved" seal on the bottle. "CL" stands for ConsumerLab.com, which is an independent supplements industry watchdog that tests the quality of supplements and gives its seal of approval only to the best.

• Choose supplements that contain minerals in chelated form. This means the minerals are attached to proteins, just as they are in real foods; this aids absorption.

• Look for enzymes in the formulation. Certain enzymes help your body absorb vitamins and minerals.

• Take your vitamin and mineral supplement with a meal. This, too, will aid absorption.

WHEY PROTEIN

Discussions about fats never fail to distinguish the different types of fat that have different effects on the body. Likewise, discussions about carbohydrates always distinguish different types of carbohydrate that have different effects in the body. But discussions about proteins almost always fail to explain that there are also different types of proteins that affect the body in different ways.

All proteins are made up of some combination of the twenty amino acids; individual proteins contain different numbers and proportions of these amino acids. In addition, protein-containing foods differ in terms of the types and amounts of proteins they contain. Thus various proteins and protein-containing foods affect the body in different ways.

Scientists have various methods of measuring protein quality. Biological value (BV) is a measure of a particular protein's effect on nitrogen balance (the more positive the better). The protein digestibility corrected amino acid score (PCDAAS) is a measure of how well a particular protein supplies the nine essential amino acids (the more completely the better). Proteins from

PHASE III

WHEY PROTEIN SUPPLEMENTS

Aria Women's Protein

CytoSport Complete Whey Protein

Designer Whey

GNC Pro Performance® 100% Whey Protein

Optimum Nutrition 100% Whey Gold Standard

animal food sources (meat, fish, eggs, dairy) have higher ratings than do plant proteins on both scales. Animal proteins are more similar to human proteins than plant proteins are. For this reason our bodies are able to make more efficient use of animal proteins. Also, unlike most animal proteins, most plant proteins contain very small amounts of, or are missing entirely, one or more of three essential amino acids: tryptophan, methionine, and lysine. This, too, makes plant proteins less effective in the body. Finally, animal foods tend to contain much larger amounts of protein than do plant foods. It's not necessary to eat animal foods to get enough of the essential amino acids. You can get all you need as a vegetarian, but it's quite a bit easier as an omnivore.

The highest-quality protein of all is whey protein, which is actually a collection of three proteins in cow's milk. Whey is isolated from milk in standard cheesemaking. Whey proteins are distilled from whey into a powder containing little or no fat and lactose (milk sugar, which some people have trouble digesting) and are used in a variety of protein supplements.

Whey protein is a complete protein that contains all nine essential amino acids. Its protein digestibility corrected amino acid score is 1.14, as compared to 0.94 for beef protein, and its biological value is an astronomical 149, compared to 100 for eggs. In addition, whey protein empties from the stomach and is absorbed into the bloodstream from the intestine faster than other proteins. Finally, whey contains especially high concentrations of amino acids that are metabolized at high rates during exercise—most notably glutamine and leucine.

Men and women can meet all of their basic protein needs without using a whey protein supplement, even as vegetarians. However, because of its unmatched quality and fast-acting nature, whey protein provides extra benefits when taken supplementally. Studies have shown that a daily whey protein supplement is a perfect complement to an exercise program in that it enhances the muscle-building effect of exercise and increases carbohydrate storage in the liver and muscles (which reduces the conversion of carbohydrates to stored fats).

There is a wide variety of whey protein supplements on the market. I recommend that you use a plain whey protein powder that you can add to smoothies or other drinks you blend or mix for yourself. Alternatively, use a post-workout recovery drink mix containing whey protein, such as Endurox R⁴ or Ultragen RS Recovery Drink. Appropriate serving sizes range from 12 to 25 grams. The smaller figure is appropriate for smaller individuals (less than 125 pounds), after lighter workouts, and for those who are not especially interested in gaining muscle mass. The larger figure is appropriate for larger individuals (more than 185 pounds), following harder workouts, and for those who are interested in gaining significant muscle mass.

Following is a summary of the nature, benefits, and recommended usage of the seven nutritional supplements I'd like you to consider trying in Phase III of the Lean Look program.

SUPPLEMENTS SUMMARY

SUPPLEMENT	WHAT IT IS	WHAT IT DOES	RECOMMENDED USAGE
Beta-alanine	Amino acid precursor of carnosine, a muscle acid buffer	Enhances high-intensity exercise performance, which in turn enhances muscle-toning and fat-burning benefits	1–4 grams daily
Creatine	Nutrient precursor of creatine phosphate, a muscle fuel	Enhances high-intensity exercise performance, which in turn enhances muscle-toning and fat-burning benefits	2.5–5 grams daily after 4- to 7-day, 20 grams/day loading period
Fish oil/ Flaxseed oil	Oils rich in omega-3 essential fatty acids	Improves cell membrane health, nerve transmission, and so forth	1,000 milligrams of omega-3 EFAs daily from food and supplements combined
Fiber	An indigestible form of complex carbohydrate	Increases fullness, reduces eating, and promotes leanness	35 grams daily total (including fiber from food and supplementation combined)
Glucosamine/ Chondroitin	Components of joint cartilage	Reduces joint pain; improves joint function	Glucosamine: 1,500 milligrams daily Chondroitin: 800 milligrams daily
Vitamin and mineral supplement	A supplement containing multiple essential vitamins and minerals	Promotes all-around health	As a general rule 50–200% USRDA of each vitamin and mineral

PHASE III

Whey Protein	A collection of three high-quality proteins extracted from whey isolated from cow's milk	Enhances muscle fueling, repair and toning; reduces fat storage	12–25 grams daily

WHAT ABOUT DIET PILLS?

Weight-loss supplements are the fastest-growing segment of the multibillion-dollar nutritional supplements industry. Despite the popularity of weight-loss supplements and the great variety of such products on the market, not a single one of them has yet proven to be safe and effective for the long term. I don't deny the possibility that a safe and effective supplement for weight loss or weight control might be developed one day—again, I let science guide my beliefs about nutrition, not ideology—but that day has not yet come.

The apparent variety of weight-loss supplements is somewhat illusory. Many weight-loss formulas contain the same ingredients (most of which are stimulants). Following is a list of ingredients to watch out for and avoid in many popular weight-loss supplements.

Bitter orange. A stimulant (also known as citrus aurantium) that artificially revs up the nervous system, bitter orange became a popular ingredient in diet products after ephedra was banned by the Food and Drug Administration. The active chemical in bitter orange is synephrine, which is very similar to ephedra. Bitter orange is associated with similar side effects (increased risk of high blood pressure, heart attack, and stroke) while being less effective for weight loss. CortiSlim and Ripped Fuel contain bitter orange.

Caffeine. Also a stimulant, caffeine may facilitate weight loss by boosting activity levels. Caffeine is acceptable in small amounts, but many diet products contain large amounts of caffeine, which are associated with side effects including jitters and insomnia. ThermaLean-RX, Lipovarin, and Zantrex 3 contain large amounts of caffeine.

Chitosan. A type of fiber that is derived from the shells of crustaceans, chitosan (pronounced *ky-to-san)* absorbs dietary fats and oils and prevents them from being stored in the body. Chitosan proponents claim this action facilitates weight loss. While chitosan supplementation does appear to cause a mild reduction in LDL cholesterol, research does not support the weight-loss claim. Side effects include gas, bloating, and diarrhea. Advaslim contains chitosan.

Chromium. An essential trace mineral (i.e., a mineral humans need in very small amounts), chromium is naturally present in foods such as beef, eggs, and spinach. It is also an ingredient in many diet products because it is known to assist naturally in the metabolism of carbs and fats, as well as in blood sugar regulation. There is no evidence, however, that chromium supplementation facilitates weight loss. Hydroxycut contains chromium.

Garcinia. An extract from the fruit of the garcinia tree is used in several diet products. The main active compound in garcinia fruit extract is hydroxicitric acid (HCA). Proponents of HCA claim that it promotes weight loss by suppressing appetite and preventing the conversion of dietary carbohydrates to fats. However, a recent review of studies on HCA published in the *Journal of the American Medical Association* concluded that HCA is ineffective in promoting weight loss. Garcinia fruit extract is the main active ingredient in Citrimax.

Hoodia gordonii. This herbal extract from a species of cactus has been the subject of a lot of recent hype. Yet only one poorly designed study has shown any weight-loss benefit, and it involved doses many times greater than can be found in any commercially available product. Hoodia gordonii is the active ingredient in Trimspa (recently fined by the Federal Trade Commission for making false claims).

7-Keto. This chemical is derived from DHEA. A steroid prohormone, DHEA was once promoted as a miracle weight-loss product until studies showed it had limited effectiveness and may increase the risk of cardiovascular disease. Lean System 7 and Lipovarin contain 7-keto.

Perhaps someday achieving the Lean Look will be as easy as taking a pill. But until that day comes, it is important to avoid falling into the "magic bullet" mentality. Nothing works if you don't. The Lean Look is simply impossible to achieve without a healthy diet and regular exercise. As an adjunct to these good habits, a few key nutritional supplements can take your leanness and overall health one step further.

CHAPTER 14

Resistance Exercise: Power Development

Most athletes and exercisers are familiar with the idea that the effects of resistance workouts are influenced by factors such as the load, or resistance level, the number of repetitions, and the number of sets. For example, you probably know that heavy loads and fewer repetitions build more muscle mass, while higher repetitions with lighter loads develop more muscular endurance. But many athletes and exercisers overlook the fact that the *speed* of repetitions also affects how your muscles respond to resistance workouts. In other words, doing slow lifts has a different effect than doing fast lifts.

Go to any gym and you'll see that almost everyone there does slow lifts exclusively. There's nothing wrong with slow lifts, but fast lifts have their place too. When you combine a moderate load with fast repetitions, the primary conditioning effect is power development. Power—the combination of strength and speed—is a crucial capacity in virtually every sport, so I do a lot of power work with my competitive athletes. Power-development exercises are beneficial for noncompetitive athletes as well; by challenging your muscles in a somewhat different way than they are accustomed to, these exercises promote further development even after you have laid a solid fitness foundation. In addition, increasing your muscle power will help you perform your cardio intervals at a higher level and get more out of them. Also the variation keeps things interesting!

One of my current clients is Megan, a twenty-four-year-old special needs teacher and waitress. I put her on a version of the Lean Look program that was tailored to fit her particular situation, which included an irregular daily schedule and a background as a competitive volleyball player. Megan responded well to all aspects of the Lean Look program, including high-intensity cardio intervals, nutrient timing, and circuit resistance workouts, but she responded especially well to the power training workouts that I'm about to show you. They helped her gain strength and reshape her body quickly, helping her reduce her body fat from 20 percent to 17 percent—enough to make an obvious improvement in her physique—in only ten weeks.

In Phase III you will perform one power workout each week along with two strength-building workouts of the sort you did in Phase II. In this chapter I will present a number of power exercises that you will use in your power-development workouts. You can also convert many of the muscle-balancing exercises described in chapter 6 and many of the strength-building exercises described in chapter 10 into power exercises by doing them faster and adjusting the level of resistance. Not every muscle-balancing or strength-building exercise can be done safely or effectively at a fast tempo, but many can. The new exercises in this chapter and the convertible exercises from Phase I and Phase II will combine to give you an ample pool of exercises to choose from in creating power workouts.

The chart that follows lists 22 muscle-balancing and strength-building exercises from chapters 6 and 10 that can be converted to power development exercises by speeding up the repetitions. The word *power* is incorporated into the name of each exercise to distinguish it from the original version.

MUSCLE-BALANCING AND STRENGTH-BUILDING RESISTANCE EXERCISES THAT CAN BE CONVERTED TO POWER DEVELOPMENT RESISTANCE EXERCISES

EXERCISE	SEE PAGE	CATEGORY	EQUIPMENT REQUIRED	MUSCLES TARGETED
Heel Raise → Power Heel Raise	70	Legs	Exercise bench (dumbbells optional)	Calves
Weighted Heel Raise → Power Weighted Heel Raise	155	Legs	Dumbbells	Calves
Heel Dip → Power Heel Dip	72	Legs	Stair step	Calves
Double-Leg Buck → Power Double-Leg Buck	73	Legs	Exercise bench or chair	Hamstrings
Squat with Dumbbells → Power Squat	151	Legs	Dumbbells	Hips, quadriceps, hamstrings, buttocks
Forward Lunge → Power Lunge	152	Legs	None	Hamstrings, quadriceps, buttocks
Lying Hip Adduction → Power Lying Hip Adduction	68	Legs	None	Hips
Dumbbell Row → Power Dumbbell Row	74	Core	Dumbbells	Mid-back
Weighted Sit-up → Power Weighted Sit-up	158	Core	Any type of weight	Outer abs
Reverse Crunch → Power Reverse Crunch	163	Core	None	Lower abs
Cable Pull-down → Power Cable Pull-down	75	Core	Cable pull-down	Mid-back
Oblique Crunch → Power Oblique Crunch	77	Core	None	Outer abs, obliques

PHASE III

Crunch Twist → Power Crunch Twist	162	Core	None	Outer abs, obliques
Shoulder Press → Power Shoulder Press	83	Upper body	Dumbbells	Rear shoulders
Push-up → Power Push-up	85	Upper body	None	Chest, rear shoulders
Dumbbell Flye → Power Dumbbell Flye	82	Upper body	Exercise bench, dumbbells	Chest
Cable Side Shoulder Raise → Power Cable Side Shoulder Raise	87	Upper body	Cable resistance	Mid-shoulders
Biceps Curl → Power Biceps Curl	169	Upper body	Dumbbells	Biceps
Cable Front Shoulder Raise → Power Cable Front Shoulder Raise	88	Upper body	Cable resistance	Front shoulders
Triceps Press → Power Triceps Press	171	Upper body	Dumbbells	Triceps
Upright Cable Row → Power Upright Cable Row	89	Upper body	Cable resistance	Upper back
Standing Single-Arm Cable Flye → Power Standing Single-Arm Cable Flye	166	Upper body	Cable resistance	Chest

As you may have noticed in looking over this list, more cable exercises than dumbbell exercises are convertible to power exercises. This is because not as many dumbbell exercises can be done safely at a fast tempo. Even so, you can easily do a complete power workout without the use of cable resistance. Three of the exercises (Push-up, Oblique Crunch, and Crunch Twist) listed in the table do not involve cables or any other equipment, and 6 of the 9 new exercises presented later in this chapter do not require cables.

To convert any of the exercises listed in the table to a power excrcise, simply perform both the lifting and lowering segments of the exercises at twice the tempo you would normally do them without any pause between lifting and lowering. Do not rush or flail—just go faster. Be especially careful when performing the lowering segment of dumbbell exercises such as the Shoulder Press at a fast tempo. It's important that you do not let the weights simply drop toward your body. Resist gravity as you do when performing the exercise at a moderate tempo, but resist it somewhat less, so that the weights move downward more quickly, yet still under control.

For non–body weight exercises, choose a resistance that you can lift 12 times at this high tempo. If you can do 12 lifts, but not without slowing down toward the end of the set, the resistance is too high. You will not get the same power-building benefit if you go past the point where you have to begin slowing down due to fatigue. To ensure that you don't slow down, use the plus-one rule: that is, choose a resistance level that you're pretty sure you could lift 13 times before slowing down, even though you actually lift it only 12 times in the workout. For body weight exercises, do as many repetitions as you can without slowing down, minus one, up to a maximum of 15 repetitions.

POWER DEVELOPMENT EXERCISES

Here are the 9 new exercises that are power exercises through and through—3 exercises for the legs, 3 for the core, and 3 for the upper body.

LEG EXERCISES

You will notice that the leg exercises are all jumping movements. Jumping movements are inherently power exercises because they require high-speed, high-intensity muscle contractions.

Scissor Jump

MUSCLES TARGETED: thighs, buttocks, hips, calves

EQUIPMENT REQUIRED: none

Stand with your left foot half a step ahead of your right foot and both knees bent. Now leap as high off the floor as you can. While in the air, reverse the position of your feet so that when you land your right foot is a half step ahead of your left. Immediately lower yourself into another deep squat. Complete 16 to 24 jumps (8 to 12 in each position).

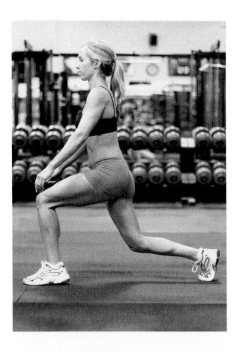
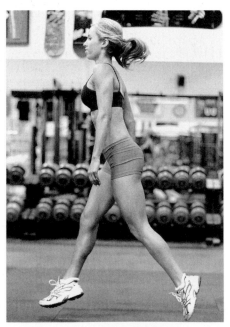

Single-Leg Box Jump

MUSCLES TARGETED: hips, buttocks, thighs, calves

EQUIPMENT REQUIRED: aerobic step or regular stair step

Balance on your left foot facing a sturdy platform (such as an exercise step) that is 10 to 18 inches in height. Leap up onto the platform, landing on your left foot, and immediately leap back down to the floor. Do 12 repetitions and then switch to the right foot.

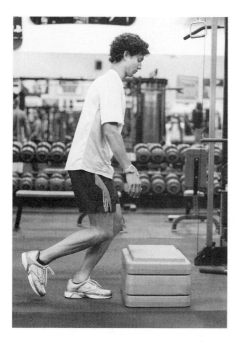 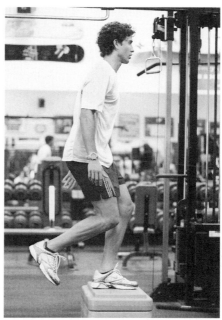

Wall Jump

MUSCLES TARGETED: calves

EQUIPMENT REQUIRED: none

Stand facing a wall with your nose just a few inches away from it. Extend your arms straight overhead. Jump as high as you can without bending your knees, so that all of your power is coming from your calf muscles. Touch your fingers to the highest point you can reach. Land on your forefeet and immediately jump again without letting your heels touch the ground. You're essentially bouncing on your forefeet. Continue for 20 to 30 seconds.

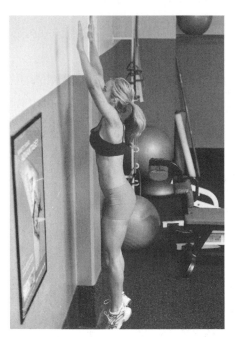 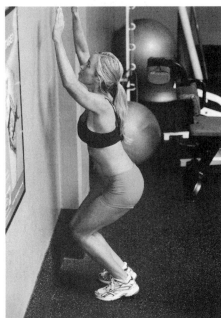

CORE EXERCISES

Following are three power development resistance exercises for the core.

Tuck Jump

MUSCLES TARGETED: abs, hip flexors, thighs, calves

EQUIPMENT REQUIRED: none

Begin in a normal standing position. Bend both legs slightly and leap as high as you can. As you approach the apex of your flight, pull your knees up to your chest. Quickly extend your legs again before landing. Jump 12 to 20 times.

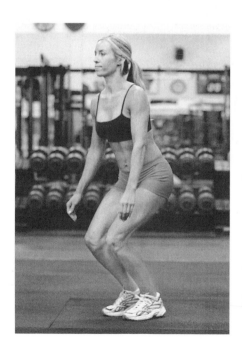
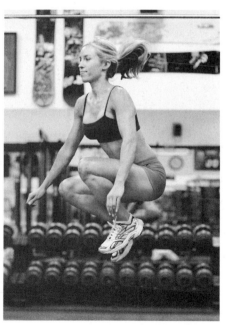

Standing One-Arm Cable Pulldown

MUSCLES TARGETED: abs, obliques, shoulders

EQUIPMENT REQUIRED: cable resistance

Stand facing a cable pulley station or door gym with a handle attached above head height. Using an overhand grip, grasp the handle with your left hand. With a smooth, powerful movement, pull the handle down toward the floor, keeping your arm straight. Return to the starting position. Do 12 repetitions and then repeat the exercise using your right hand.

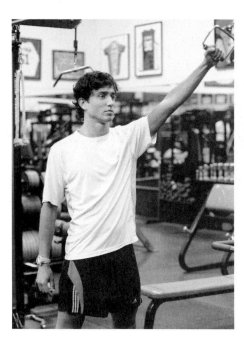 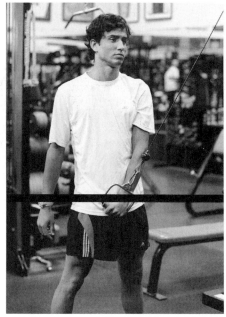

Mountain Climber

MUSCLES TARGETED: abs, hip flexors

EQUIPMENT REQUIRED: none

Assume a push-up position with your right leg sharply bent and your right foot positioned midway between your left foot and right hand, forefoot on the floor, heel up. Now switch the positions of your legs as quickly as possible, drawing your left knee powerfully forward toward your chest and kicking powerfully backward with your right leg. Continue switching your legs back and forth for 20 to 30 seconds.

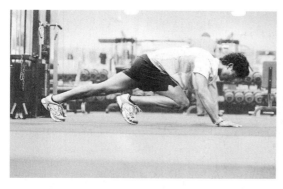 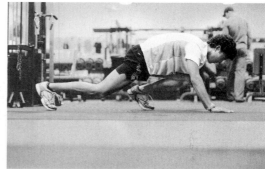

UPPER BODY EXERCISES

Following are three power development resistance exercises for the upper body.

One-Arm Dumbbell Snatch

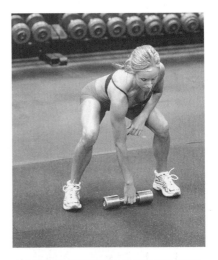

MUSCLES TARGETED: shoulders, upper back, lower back, buttocks, legs

EQUIPMENT REQUIRED: dumbbell

Assume a wide athletic stance with a single dumbbell placed on the floor between your feet. Bend your knees, tilt forward from the hips, and grasp the dumbbell with your right hand. Begin with your right arm fully extended. With a single, fluid, powerful movement, yank the dumbbell off the floor, stand fully upright, and continue raising your right arm until it is extended straight overhead. (Bend your arm as necessary to keep the dumbbell close to your body so that it travels upward in a straight line.) Pause briefly and then reverse the movement, allowing the dumbbell to come to rest again on the floor briefly before initiating the next lift. Complete 12 repetitions and then switch to the left arm. This exercise can be done with a kettlebell, if the gym where you workout has kettlebells available. (A kettlebell looks like a metal candlepin bowling ball with a handle.)

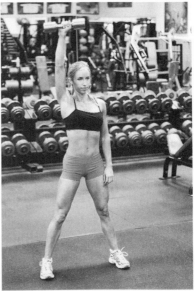

Incline Power Push-up

MUSCLES TARGETED: chest, shoulders, upper back, triceps

EQUIPMENT REQUIRED: exercise bench

Assume a push-up position with your hands resting not on the floor but on a stable support such as an exercise bench. The shorter the support is, the more challenging this exercise becomes. Bend your arms until your chest comes within an inch or two of the bench. With a fluid, powerful motion, extend your arms and thrust as far away from the support as you can. Maintain a rigid, straight line with your body throughout this movement. As your hands come back into contact with the support, immediately lower your chest toward it to prepare for the next thrust. Complete as many power push-ups as you can without slowing down, up to a maximum of 20. For a greater challenge, clap your hands together during the "floating" phase of the power push-up.

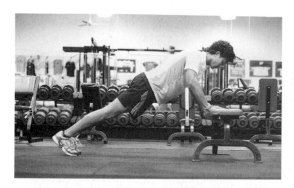
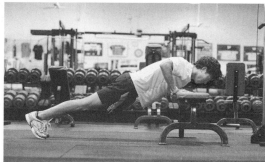
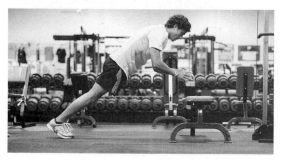

Reverse Wood Chop

MUSCLES TARGETED: shoulders, upper back, lower back, obliques, hips

EQUIPMENT REQUIRED: cable resistance

Connect a handle to the low attachment point of a door gym or cable pulley station. Stand in a wide stance with your left side facing the door gym or cable pulley station and most of your weight on the left foot. Grasp the handle in both hands, beginning with the handle just outside your left knee. Using both arms, pull the cable upward and across your body, finishing above your right shoulder. Avoid rounding your back. Return smoothly to the start position. Complete 12 repetitions and then switch sides.

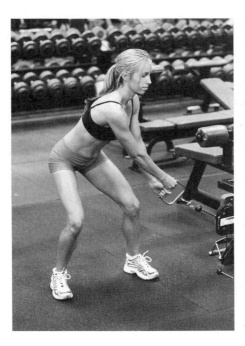
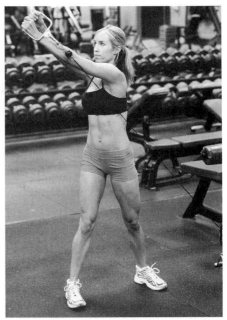

The following table provides summary information about all 9 of the specific power-development exercises presented in this chapter. These 9 exercises, in addition to the 22 convertible exercises summarized in Table 14.1, represent the total pool of power-development exercises you can use to create power-development resistance workouts for use in Phase III of the Lean Look program.

SUMMARY OF SPECIFIC POWER DEVELOPMENT RESISTANCE EXERCISES

EXERCISE	TYPE	EQUIPMENT	MUSCLES TARGETED
Scissor Jump	Legs	None	Thighs, buttocks, hips, calves
Single-Leg Box Jump	Legs	Aerobic step or regulare stair step	Hips, buttocks, thighs, calves
Wall Jump	Legs	None	Calves
Tuck Jump	Core	None	Abs, hip flexors, thighs, calves
Standing One-Arm Cable Pull-down	Core	Cable resistance	Abs, obliques, shoulders
Mountain Climber	Core	None	Abs, hip flexors
One-Arm Dumbbell Snatch	Upper body	Dumbbell	Shoulders, upper back, lower back, buttocks, legs
Incline Power Push-up	Upper body	Exercise bench	Chest, shoulders, upper back, triceps
Reverse Wood Chop	Upper body	Cable resistance	Shoulders, upper back, lower back, obliques, hips

POWER-DEVELOPMENT RESISTANCE WORKOUT GUIDELINES

Your power-development resistance workouts will be circuit workouts with the same structure as your muscle-balancing and strength-building workouts. Each workout will consist of 9 or 12 total exercises, or three or four sets of a legs exercise, followed by a core exercise, and an upper body exercise. Within these parameters, feel free to choose and arrange power exercises from the lists of options presented on pages 221 and 233 as you see fit. Note that the new exercises described in the preceding section comprise a complete power workout that you can use as a starting point. You may substitute one or more of the convertible exercises listed in the chart on page 221 for the specific power-development exercises according to equipment constraints or any other factor, and you may add exercises from those listed in this chart to the sequence of specific power-development exercises to create a 12-exercise power workout. If you prefer not to design your own power-development resistance workouts, just choose the appropriate ready-made power-development workout from the last section of this chapter.

One important difference between power-development resistance workouts and muscle-balancing and strength-building resistance workouts is that they call for a little more rest time between exercises. The speed factor greatly increases the total energy demand of power-development exercises. Consequently, when you complete a power exercise you will probably find yourself more out of breath and will therefore need more time to regain control of your breathing. We strength and conditioning coaches refer to this phenomenon as *oxygen deficit,* or *excess postexercise oxygen consumption* (EPOC). It happens because oxygen is needed to clean up the metabolic by-products of anaerobic energy release in the muscles. Since power exercises generally require more anaerobic energy, they produce more of these by-products, which your body must process before your muscles are ready to perform again at the same level.

When doing power workouts you should take the minimum amount of rest time between exercises that you need to do the next exercise at the same level. You will probably find that you need at least 30–45 seconds. At first you may need to experiment with various rest times to determine which is truly the minimum needed. Before long you'll get a feel for it. By paying attention to your breathing and the sensations within your muscles you will know when they have recovered sufficiently to perform the next exercise at the desired level.

READY-MADE POWER-DEVELOPMENT RESISTANCE CIRCUITS

The charts that follow present ready-made power-development resistance circuits to use in Phase III. There are two beginner circuits (consisting of 9 exercises) and two advanced circuits (consisting of 12 exercises). One of each of the beginner and advanced circuits requires no equipment other than cable resistance. The other circuits require only an exercise bench and dumbbells.

These ready-made circuits do not represent complete workouts. You will repeat your chosen circuit two or three times as prescribed in the Phase III resistance workout schedules at the end of the chapter.

BEGINNER POWER-DEVELOPMENT RESISTANCE CIRCUIT #1 (9 EXERCISES)

Equipment: cable resistance

Leg Exercise #1	Scissor Jump (page 224)
Core Exercise #1	Tuck Jump (page 227)
Upper Body Exercise #1	Reverse Wood Chop (page 232)
Leg Exercise #2	Power Lunge (pages 152, 221)
Core Exercise #2	Mountain Climber (page 229)
Upper Body Exercise #2	Power Push-up (pages 85, 222)
Leg Exercise #3	Wall Jump (page 226)
Core Exercise #3	Power Cable Pull-down (pages 75, 221)
Upper Body Exercise #3	Power Cable Front Shoulder Raise (pages 87, 222)

BEGINNER POWER-DEVELOPMENT RESISTANCE CIRCUIT #2 (9 EXERCISES)

Equipment: exercise bench and dumbbells

Leg Exercise #1	Single-Leg Box Jump (page 225)
Core Exercise #1	Tuck Jump (page 227)
Upper Body Exercise #1	One-Arm Dumbbell Snatch (page 230)
Leg Exercise #2	Power Squat (pages 151, 221)
Core Exercise #2	Power Dumbbell Row (pages 74, 221)
Upper Body Exercise #2	Incline Power Push-up (page 231)
Leg Exercise #3	Power Weighted Heel Raise (pages 155, 221)
Core Exercise #3	Mountain Climber (page 229)
Upper Body Exercise #3	Power Triceps Press (pages 171, 222)

ADVANCED POWER-DEVELOPMENT RESISTANCE CIRCUIT #1 (12 EXERCISES)

Equipment: stability ball and cable resistance

Leg Exercise #1	Scissor Jump (page 224)
Core Exercise #1	Tuck Jump (page 227)
Upper Body Exercise #1	Reverse Wood Chop (page 232)
Leg Exercise #2	Power Lunge (pages 152, 221)
Core Exercise #2	Mountain Climber (page 229)
Upper Body Exercise #2	Power Push-up (pages 85, 222)
Leg Exercise #3	Single-Leg Box Jump (page 225)
Core Exercise #3	Power Oblique Crunch (pages 77, 221)
Upper Body Exercise #3	Power Upright Cable Row (pages 89, 222)
Leg Exercise #4	Wall Jump (page 226)
Core Exercise #4	Power Cable Pull-down (pages 75, 221)
Upper Body Exercise #4	Power Cable Front Shoulder Raise (page 88)

ADVANCED POWER-DEVELOPMENT RESISTANCE CIRCUIT #2 (12 EXERCISES)

Equipment: exercise bench and dumbbells

Leg Exercise #1	Single-Leg Box Jump (page 225)
Core Exercise #1	Tuck Jump (page 227)
Upper Body Exercise #1	One-Arm Dumbbell Snatch (page 230)
Leg Exercise #2	Power Squat (pages 151, 221)
Core Exercise #2	Power Dumbbell Row (pages 74, 221)
Upper Body Exercise #2	Incline Power Push-up (page 231)
Leg Exercise #3	Scissor Jump (page 224)
Core Exercise #3	Power Crunch Twist (pages 77, 222)
Upper Body Exercise #3	Power Dumbbell Press (pages 83, 222)
Leg Exercise #4	Power Weighted Heel Raise (pages 155, 221)
Core Exercise #4	Mountain Climber (page 229)
Upper Body Exercise #4	Power Triceps Press (pages 171, 222)

DETAILED PHASE III RESISTANCE WORKOUT SCHEDULES

The following charts present detailed Phase III resistance workout schedules for the beginner and advanced levels. Throughout this phase you will do power-development resistance workouts on Wednesday. On Monday and Friday you will continue to do a strength-building resistance workout as you did throughout Phase II.

BEGINNER

Wk #	Monday	Wednesday	Friday
9	Strength-Building Resistance Workout	Power-Development Resistance Workout	Strength-Building Resistance Workout
	Summary 2 circuits 9 exercises 21 minutes	Summary 2 circuits 9 exercises 21 minutes	Summary 2 circuits 9 exercises 21 minutes
	Workout:	Workout:	Workout:
	Warm-up	Warm-up	Warm-up
	2X Strength-Building Leg Exercise #1	2X Power Leg Exercise #1	2X Strength-Building Leg Exercise #1
	Strength-Building Core Exercise #1	Power Core Exercise #1	Strength-Building Core Exercise #1
	Strength-Building Upper Body Exercise #1	Power Upper Body Exercise #1	Strength-Building Upper Body Exercise #1
	Strength-Building Leg Exercise #2	Power Leg Exercise #2	Strength-Building Leg Exercise #2
	Strength-Building Core Exercise #2	Power Core Exercise #2	Strength-Building Core Exercise #2
	Strength-Building Upper Body Exercise #2	Power Upper Body Exercise #2	Strength-Building Upper Body Exercise #2
	Strength-Building Leg Exercise #3	Power Leg Exercise #3	Strength-Building Leg Exercise #3
	Strength-Building Core Exercise #3	Power Core Exercise #3	Strength-Building Core Exercise #3
	Strength-Building Upper Body Exercise #3	Power Upper Body Exercise #3	Strength-Building Upper Body Exercise #3

Wk #	Monday	Wednesday	Friday
10	Strength-Building Resistance Workout	Power-Development Resistance Workout	Strength-Building Resistance Workout
	Summary 3 circuits 9 exercises 30 minutes	Summary 3 circuits 9 exercises 30 minutes	Summary 3 circuits 9 exercises 30 minutes
	Workout:	Workout:	Workout:
	Warm-up	Warm-up	Warm-up
	3X Strength-Building Leg Exercise #1	3X Power Leg Exercise #1	3X Strength-Building Leg Exercise #1
	Strength-Building Core Exercise #1	Power Core Exercise #1	Strength-Building Core Exercise #1
	Strength-Building Upper Body Exercise #1	Power Upper Body Exercise #1	Strength-Building Upper Body Exercise #1
	Strength-Building Leg Exercise #2	Power Leg Exercise #2	Strength-Building Leg Exercise #2
	Strength-Building Core Exercise #2	Power Core Exercise #2	Strength-Building Core Exercise #2
	Strength-Building Upper Body Exercise #2	Power Upper Body Exercise #2	Strength-Building Upper Body Exercise #2
	Strength-Building Leg Exercise #3	Power Leg exercise #3	Strength-Building Leg Exercise #3
	Strength-Building Core Exercise #3	Power Core Exercise #3	Strength-Building Core Exercise #3
	Strength-Building Upper Body Exercise #3	Power Upper Body Exercise #3	Strength-Building Upper Body Exercise #3

The beginner and advanced schedules are the same in Phase III except that the advanced workouts include 12 exercises per circuit while the beginner workouts include only 9 exercises per circuit.

Wk #	Monday	Wednesday	Friday
11	Strength-Building Resistance Workout	Power-Development Resistance Workout	Strength-Building Resistance Workout
	Summary 3 circuits 9 exercises 30 minutes	Summary 3 circuits 9 exercises 30 minutes	Summary 3 circuits 9 exercises 30 minutes
	Workout:	Workout:	Workout:
	Warm-up	Warm-up	Warm-up
	3X Strength-Building Leg Exercise #1	3X Power Leg Exercise #1	3X Strength-Building Leg Exercise #1
	Strength-Building Core Exercise #1	Power Core Exercise #1	Strength-Building Core Exercise #1
	Strength-Building Upper Body Exercise #1	Power Upper Body Exercise #1	Strength-Building Upper Body Exercise #1
	Strength-Building Leg Exercise #2	Power Leg Exercise #2	Strength-Building Leg Exercise #2
	Strength-Building Core Exercise #2	Power Core Exercise #2	Strength-Building Core Exercise #2
	Strength-Building Upper Body Exercise #2	Power Upper Body Exercise #2	Strength-Building Upper Body Exercise #2
	Strength-Building Leg Exercise #3	Power Leg Exercise #3	Strength-Building Leg Exercise #3
	Strength-Building Core Exercise #3	Power Core Exercise #3	Strength-Building Core Exercise #3
	Strength-Building Upper Body Exercise #3	Power Upper Body Exercise #3	Strength-Building Upper Body Exercise #3

PHASE III

239

Wk #	Monday	Wednesday	Friday
12	Strength-Building Resistance Workout	Power-Development Resistance Workout	Strength-Building Resistance Workout
	Summary 2 circuits 9 exercises 21 minutes	Summary 2 circuits 9 exercises 21 minutes	Summary 2 circuits 9 exercises 21 minutes
	Workout:	Workout:	Workout:
	Warm-up	Warm-up	Warm-up
	2X Strength-Building Leg Exercise #1	2X Power Leg Exercise #1	2X Strength-Building Leg Exercise #1
	Strength-Building Core Exercise #1	Power Core Exercise #1	Strength-Building Core Exercise #1
	Strength-Building Upper Body Exercise #1	Power Upper Body Exercise #1	Strength-Building Upper Body Exercise #1
	Strength-Building Leg Exercise #2	Power Leg Exercise #2	Strength-Building Leg Exercise #2
	Strength-Building Core Exercise #2	Power Core Exercise #2	Strength-Building Core Exercise #2
	Strength-Building Upper Body Exercise #2	Power Upper Body Exercise #2	Strength-Building Upper Body Exercise #2
	Strength-Building Leg Exercise #3	Power Leg Exercise #3	Strength-Building Leg Exercise #3
	Strength-Building Core Exercise #3	Power Core Exercise #3	Strength-Building Core Exercise #3
	Strength-Building Upper Body Exercise #3	Power Upper Body Exercise #3	Strength-Building Upper Body Exercise #3

ADVANCED SCHEDULE

Wk #	Monday	Wednesday	Friday
9	Strength-Building Resistance Workout	Power-Development Resistance Workout	Strength-Building Resistance Workout
	Summary 2 circuits 12 exercises 27 minutes	Summary 2 circuits 12 exercises 27 minutes	Summary 2 circuits 12 exercises 27 minutes
	Workout:	Workout:	Workout:
	Warm-up	Warm-up	Warm-up
	2X Strength-Building Leg Exercise #1	2X Power Leg Exercise #1	2X Strength-Building Leg Exercise #1
	Strength-Building Core Exercise #1	Power Core Exercise #1	Strength-Building Core Exercise #1
	Strength-Building Upper Body Exercise #1	Power Upper Body Exercise #1	Strength-Building Upper Body Exercise #1
	Strength-Building Leg Exercise #2	Power Leg Exercise #2	Strength-Building Leg Exercise #2
	Strength-Building Core Exercise #2	Power Core Exercise #2	Strength-Building Core Exercise #2
	Strength-Building Upper Body Exercise #2	Power Upper Body Exercise #2	Strength-Building Upper Body Exercise #2
	Strength-Building Leg Exercise #3	Power Leg Exercise #3	Strength-Building Leg Exercise #3
	Strength-Building Core Exercise #3	Power Core Exercise #3	Strength-Building Core Exercise #3
	Strength-Building Upper Body Exercise #3	Power Upper Body Exercise #3	Strength-Building Upper Body Exercise #3
	Strength-Building Leg Exercise #4	Power Leg Exercise #4	Strength-Building Leg Exercise #4
	Strength-Building Core Exercise #4	Power Core Exercise #4	Strength-Building Core Exercise #4
	Strength-Building Upper Body Exercise #4	Power Upper Body Exercise #4	Strength-Building Upper Body Exercise #4

Wk #	Monday	Wednesday	Friday
10	Strength-Building Resistance Workout	Power-Development Resistance Workout	Strength-Building Resistance Workout
	Summary 3 circuits 12 exercises 39 minutes	Summary 3 circuits 12 exercises 39 minutes	Summary 3 circuits 12 exercises 39 minutes
	Workout:	Workout:	Workout:
	Warm-up	Warm-up	Warm-up
	3X Strength-Building Leg Exercise #1	3X Power Leg Exercise #1	3X Strength-Building Leg Exercise #1
	Strength-Building Core Exercise #1	Power Core Exercise #1	Strength-Building Core Exercise #1
	Strength-Building Upper Body Exercise #1	Power Upper Body Exercise #1	Strength-Building Upper Body Exercise #1
	Strength-Building Leg Exercise #2	Power Leg Exercise #2	Strength-Building Leg Exercise #2
	Strength-Building Core Exercise #2	Power Core Exercise #2	Strength-Building Core Exercise #2
	Strength-Building Upper Body Exercise #2	Power Upper Body Exercise #2	Strength-Building Upper Body Exercise #2
	Strength-Building Leg Exercise #3	Power Leg Exercise #3	Strength-Building Leg Exercise #3
	Strength-Building Core Exercise #3	Power Core Exercise #3	Strength-Building Core Exercise #3
	Strength-Building Upper Body Exercise #3	Power Upper Body Exercise #3	Strength-Building Upper Body Exercise #3
	Strength-Building Leg Exercise #4	Power Leg Exercise #4	Strength-Building Leg Exercise #4
	Strength-Building Core Exercise #4	Power Core Exercise #4	Strength-Building Core Exercise #4
	Strength-Building Upper Body Exercise #4	Power Upper Body Exercise #4	Strength-Building Upper Body Exercise #4

Wk #	Monday	Wednesday	Friday
11	Strength-Building Resistance Workout	Power-Development Resistance Workout	Strength-Building Resistance Workout
	Summary 3 circuits 12 exercises 39 minutes	Summary 3 circuits 12 exercises 39 minutes	Summary 3 circuits 12 exercises 39 minutes
	Workout:	Workout:	Workout:
	Warm-up	Warm-up	Warm-up
	3X Strength-Building Leg Exercise #1	3X Power Leg Exercise #1	3X Strength-Building Leg Exercise #1
	Strength-Building Core Exercise #1	Power Core Exercise #1	Strength-Building Core Exercise #1
	Strength-Building Upper Body Exercise #1	Power Upper Body Exercise #1	Strength-Building Upper Body Exercise #1
	Strength-Building Leg Exercise #2	Power Leg Exercise #2	Strength-Building Leg Exercise #2
	Strength-Building Core Exercise #2	Power Core Exercise #2	Strength-Building Core Exercise #2
	Strength-Building Upper Body Exercise #2	Power Upper Body Exercise #2	Strength-Building Upper Body Exercise #2
	Strength-Building Leg Exercise #3	Power Leg Exercise #3	Strength-Building Leg Exercise #3
	Strength-Building Core Exercise #3	Power Core Exercise #3	Strength-Building Core Exercise #3
	Strength-Building Upper Body Exercise #3	Power Upper Body Exercise #3	Strength-Building Upper Body Exercise #3
	Strength-Building Leg Exercise #4	Power Leg Exercise #4	Strength-Building Leg Exercise #4
	Strength-Building Core Exercise #4	Power Core Exercise #4	Strength-Building Core Exercise #4
	Strength-Building Upper Body Exercise #4	Power Upper Body Exercise #4	Strength-Building Upper Body Exercise #4

PHASE III

Wk #	Monday	Wednesday	Friday
12	Strength-Building Resistance Workout Summary 2 circuits 12 exercises 27 minutes Workout: Warm-up 2X Strength-Building Leg Exercise #1 Strength-Building Core Exercise #1 Strength-Building Upper Body Exercise #1 Strength-Building Leg Exercise #2 Strength-Building Core Exercise #2 Strength-Building Upper Body Exercise #2 Strength-Building Leg Exercise #3 Strength-Building Core Exercise #3 Strength-Building Upper Body Exercise #3 Strength-Building Leg Exercise #4 Strength-Building Core Exercise #4 Strength-Building Upper Body Exercise #4	Power-Development Resistance Workout Summary 2 circuits 12 exercises 27 minutes Workout: Warm-up 2X Power Leg Exercise #1 Power Core Exercise #1 Power Upper Body Exercise #1 Power Leg Exercise #2 Power Core Exercise #2 Power Upper Body Exercise #2 Power Leg Exercise #3 Power Core Exercise #3 Power Upper Body Exercise #3 Power Leg Exercise #4 Power Core Exercise #4 Power Upper Body Exercise #4	Strength-Building Resistance Workout Summary 2 circuits 12 exercises 27 minutes Workout: Warm-up 2X Strength-Building Leg Exercise #1 Strength-Building Core Exercise #1 Strength-Building Upper Body Exercise #1 Strength-Building Leg Exercise #2 Strength-Building Core Exercise #2 Strength-Building Upper Body Exercise #2 Strength-Building Leg Exercise #3 Strength-Building Core Exercise #3 Strength-Building Upper Body Exercise #3 Strength-Building Leg Exercise #4 Strength-Building Core Exercise #4 Strength-Building Upper Body Exercise #4

CHAPTER 15

Cardio Exercise:

Long Intervals

How do you think Lance Armstrong trained for his amazing streak of seven consecutive victories in the Tour de France? Do you think he just hopped on the bike and toured around for hours at a steady, comfortable pace every day? Not a chance! Sure, he did some steady, comfortable rides, but he also did a ton of intervals.

All competitive endurance athletes, including cyclists, runners, and swimmers, do different types of interval workouts in different phases of their training. In the early portion of the training process they usually focus on doing very short, very high intensity intervals. Then they transition to somewhat longer, slightly less intense intervals as the racing season begins. Finally, they do their longest intervals in the peak phase of their training and racing. These longer intervals are done at an intensity level that's pretty close to the intensity of their races.

Interval training was not always the standard way to train for endurance sports. Other ways of sequencing workouts were tried but were discarded after proving less effective. Endurance athletes get the best results when they focus on the most race-specific types of workouts (i.e., workouts that simulate race intensity) toward the end of the training process, when the most important race is on the horizon. These challenging peak workouts take the athlete's fitness to its highest point. But in order to be effective these workouts must be done when the athlete has already reached a fairly high level of fitness. It's the groundwork laid by the shorter intervals that allows this to happen. As I first mentioned back in chapter 3, the practice of dividing the training process into phases is known as *periodization.*

Although you aren't training to become the next Lance Armstrong, you can take advantage of the same strategy of sequencing cardio intervals to reach peak leanness and cardiovascular health. In Phase I you did very short (20-second, 30-second, and 1-minute), high-intensity cardio intervals. In Phase II you added slightly longer (2- and 3-minute) intermediate interval workouts. Now, in Phase III, you will do even longer (4- and 6-minute) intervals. The work you've done in the first two phases has prepared you to perform these longer intervals at a high level of intensity, and as a result you will get even greater benefits from these workouts.

You will continue to perform three cardio interval workouts per week in Phase III, but whereas in Phase II you did one short interval session and two intermediate interval sessions, in Phase III you will do one intermediate interval session and two long interval sessions. On Tuesdays throughout Phase III you will do a cardio workout featuring 6-minute intervals and on Saturdays you will do a cardio workout featuring 4-minute intervals. On Thursdays you will do 2- and 3-minute intervals. As you did with short and intermediate intervals, use the plus-one rule to find the right effort level for your long intervals. For example, if you're doing four higher-intensity intervals, do each at the highest work level you could sustain through five intervals, if you had to. You should complete your fourth interval feeling fatigued, but able to do one more.

Naturally, because the intervals are longer on Tuesdays and Saturdays you will not be able to sustain such a high-intensity effort as you have done in your short and intermediate intervals, and you will not be able to sustain as much of a high-intensity work level in your 6-minute-long intervals as in your 4-minute ones. You may need to experiment a little in your first 4-minute and 6-minute interval workouts to find the work level that is right for you.

4-MINUTE INTERVALS

Warm up with 5 minutes of moderate-intensity movement in your chosen activity. Next, increase your level of effort by increasing your pace and/or resistance for 4 minutes. Use the plus-one rule to guide the level of your effort. After completing the 4-minute interval, slow back down to your warm-up level of effort for 2 minutes. Once you've completed the prescribed number of 4-minute intervals, cool down for 5 minutes. Do not perform a 2-minute active recovery following your last 4-minute interval, but instead go straight to the 5-minute cooldown. Thus, a 4-minute intervals workout featuring three intervals looks like this:

5-minute easy warm-up

4 minutes hard

2-minute active recovery

4 minutes hard

2-minute active recovery

4 minutes hard

5-minute easy cooldown

Total time: 26 minutes

6-MINUTE INTERVALS

Warm up with 5 minutes of moderate-intensity movement in your chosen activity. Next, increase your level of effort by increasing your pace and/or resistance for 6 minutes. Use the plus-one rule to guide the level of your effort.

After completing the 6-minute interval, slow back down to your warm-up effort level for 3 minutes. Once you've completed the prescribed number of 6-minute intervals, cool down for 5 minutes. Do not perform a 3-minute active recovery following your last 6-minute interval, but instead go straight to the 5-minute cooldown. Thus, a 6-minute intervals workout featuring three intervals looks like this:

5-minute easy warm-up

6 minutes hard

3-minute active recovery

6 minutes hard

3-minute active recovery

6 minutes hard

5-minute easy cooldown

Total time: 34 minutes

Continue to adapt your cardio workouts to whichever form or forms of cardio exercise you prefer. The following charts provide detailed Phase III cardio workout schedules for the beginner and advanced levels. Intervals of all three types—2-minute, 4-minute, and 6-minute intervals—are designated by the word "hard," but remember that the precise level of effort should be slightly different in each.

PHASE III CARDIO EXERCISE—BEGINNER SCHEDULE

Wk #	Tuesday	Thursday	Saturday
5	6-minute intervals 5-minute easy warm-up 2 X (6 minutes hard/ 3 minutes easy) 5-minute easy cooldown Total time: 26 minutes	2-minute untervals 5-minute easy warm-up 3 X (2 minutes hard/ 2 minutes easy) 5-minute easy cooldown Total time: 20 minutes	4-minute untervals 5-minute easy warm-up 3 X (4 minutes hard/ 2 minutes easy) 5-minute easy cooldown Total time: 26 minutes
6	6-minute intervals 5-minute easy warm-up 2 X (6 minutes hard/ 3 minutes easy) 5-minute easy cooldown Total time: 26 minutes	2-minute intervals 5-minute easy warm-up 3 X (3 minutes hard/ 3 minutes easy) 5-minute easy cooldown Total time: 25 minutes	4-minute intervals 5-minute easy warm-up 3 X (4 minutes hard/ 2 minutes easy) 5-minute easy cooldown Total time: 26 minutes
7	2-minute intervals 5-minute easy warm-up 2 X (6 minutes hard/ 3 minutes easy) 5-minute easy cooldown Total time: 25 minutes	1-minute intervals 5-minute easy warm-up 4 X (2 minutes hard/ 2 minutes easy) 5-minute easy cooldown Total time: 24 minutes	4-minute intervals 5-minute easy warm-up 3 X (4 minutes hard/ 2 minutes easy) 5-minute easy cooldown Total time: 26 minutes
8	6-minute intervals 5-minute easy warm-up 2 X (6 minutes hard/ 3 minutes easy) 5-minute easy cooldown Total time: 25 minutes	3-minute intervals 5-minute easy warm-up 3 X (3 minutes hard/ 3 minutes easy) 5-minute easy cooldown Total time: 25 minutes	4-minute intervals 5-minute easy warm-up 2 X (4 minutes hard/ 2 minutes easy) 5-minute easy cooldown Total time: 20 minutes

PHASE III

249

PHASE III CARDIO EXERCISE—ADVANCED SCHEDULE

Wk #	Tuesday	Thursday	Saturday
5	2-minute intervals 5-minute easy warm-up 3 X (6 minutes hard/ 1 minute easy) 5-minute easy cooldown Total time: 34 minutes	2-minute intervals 5-minute easy warm-up 4 X (2 minutes hard/ 2 minutes easy) 5-minute easy cooldown Total time: 24 minutes	4-minute intervals 5-minute easy warm-up 3 X (4 minutes hard/ 2 minutes easy) 5-minute easy cooldown Total time: 26 minutes
6	6-minute intervals 5-minute easy warm-up 3 X (6 minutes hard/ 3 minutes easy) 5-minute easy cooldown Total time: 34 minutes	3-minute intervals 5-minute easy warm-up 4 X (3 minutes hard/ 3 minutes easy) 5-minute easy cooldown Total time: 31 minutes	4-minute intervals 5-minute easy warm-up 4 X (4 minutes hard/ 2 minutes easy) 5-minute easy cooldown Total time: 32 minutes
7	2-minute intervals 5-minute easy warm-up 4 X (6 minutes hard/ 3 minutes easy) 5-minute easy cooldown Total time: 43 minutes	2-minute intervals 5-minute easy warm-up 5 X (2 minutes hard/ 2 minutes easy) 5-minute easy cooldown Total time: 28 minutes	4-minute intervals 5-minute easy warm-up 4 X (4 minutes hard/ 2 minutes easy) 5-minute easy cooldown Total time: 32 minutes
8	6-minute intervals 5-minute easy warm-up 3 X (6 minutes hard/ 3 minutes easy) 5-minute easy cooldown Total time: 34 minutes	3-minute intervals 5-minute easy warm-up 4 X (3 minutes hard/ 3 minutes easy) 5-minute easy cooldown Total time: 31 minutes	4-minute intervals 5-minute easy warm-up 3 X (4 minutes hard/ 2 minutes easy) 5-minute easy cooldown Total time: 26 minutes

I would like to use the remainder of this chapter to talk to you about heart rate monitors and how you may use one in the cardio portion of the Lean Look program. Until this point I have prescribed workout intensity using the plus-one rule. This way of monitoring and controlling the intensity of your cardio workouts is perfectly adequate, and you don't have to use any other method if you don't wish to. But heart rate monitoring can be an excellent complement to perceived effort, and is easier to use and more affordable than you may think.

INTENSITY BY THE NUMBERS

Monitoring your heart rate during exercise enables you to measure and control your effort to ensure you get the results you are seeking. In addition, tracking your heart rate at various levels of effort from low to maximum over time gives you feedback on your progress that is both motivational and useful for the purpose of adjusting your workout program to continue getting leaner. But the first step is to purchase the right monitor.

HEART RATE MONITOR SHOPPING

The sheer variety of heart rate monitors on the market can overwhelm the first-time buyer. But shopping for a heart rate monitor is a piece of cake, if you follow these few basic guidelines.

Start with a budget. Heart rate monitors range from less than $50 to more than $350. The primary difference between the cheaper units and the costlier ones is in the number of features. Factors such as weight, materials, and durability are quite uniform across all price points.

Less can be more. Monitors with fewer buttons and features are more user-friendly, but they have some limitations. A one-button monitor, for instance, usually lacks the stopwatch functions and workout data storage capabilities of monitors with more buttons.

Know how you'll use it. The exact features you need depend on how you intend to use your monitor. For instance, if running is your favorite form of cardio exercise and you'd like to be able to monitor your pace and distance as well as your heart rate, you'll want to get a device such as the Garmin Forerunner 305, which offers both a heart rate monitor and GPS technology that enables you to measure your distance and pace in real time. But if you don't need these extra features you should stick with a simpler unit, since the Garmin Forerunner 305 costs in excess of $300.

A backlight is an important feature to have if you plan to use your monitor at night or in darkened indoor environments. Go for water resistance if you plan to use your monitor in the water. Cyclists can purchase heart rate monitors that also function as bike computers, and so forth.

Consider the future. While it's wise to buy the simplest monitor that meets your current needs, you may want to go for one or two extra features that you will likely use down the road. Sometimes people underbuy and find that they "outgrow" their monitor very quickly. Once you select a unit that you think is right, take a look at the unit above it in price and see whether it has any additional features you're likely to grow into.

BASIC TRAINING

All too often those who buy a suitable heart rate monitor never tap into its full potential or they get frustrated with simple problems such as not being able to get the darn thing started, and they end up tossing it into a drawer. To get the most out of a heart rate monitor you need to learn how to use it properly. Don't worry—it's not difficult.

The first step toward getting the most from your monitor is to read the directions. Perhaps this point sounds too obvious, but you'd be surprised by how many people purchase a monitor and then ignore the manual. So spend an hour reading the manual—it's worth every minute. With the manual in front of you, move on to the following steps:

Get familiar with the monitor. Most heart rate monitors have two basic parts: a transmitter contained within a strap worn around the chest and a display unit worn as a watch on the wrist. The transmitter reads your heart rate and feeds the information to the display unit, which gives you a readout in real time. (There are some new monitors on the market, such as the Reebok Strapless Heart Rate Monitor, that combine the transmitter and display within the wrist unit. However, there's some controversy regarding whether these devices are as accurate as traditional heart rate monitors with a chest strap.)

The simplest heart rate monitor display units have just one button that you press to start and stop the reading function. Many models also incorporate a stopwatch, which is useful when you want to time your intervals or you want to know how long it takes you to cover a measured distance. The most advanced units have four or five buttons that operate a dozen or more features. Play around with your monitor's buttons to get a sense of what they do before you use the device in a workout.

Put it on. To ensure an accurate reading, wet the sensor pads on the chest strap before you put them on. Water will do, but you can also buy special electrode gels, such as Lectron II, that work even better because they are specially formulated to conduct electrical currents and they're more viscous, so they stay between the sensor and your skin. These products are available from many heart rate monitor retailers. If you've ever worn a heart rate monitor and been unable to get a heart rate reading to come up on the display, it's likely because you didn't properly wet the sensor. This is a common oversight that stalls many a beginning heart rate monitor user right at the starting line.

Adjust the chest strap around the ribs so it fits snugly, yet comfortably, just underneath your breasts (or for men, right underneath the bulges of your chest muscles) and center the sensor over your sternum. Many first-time users find the chest strap uncomfortable. This is normal and will not last beyond the third or fourth use. I've never worked with anyone who did not eventually get used to wearing the strap. (Polar brand heart rate monitors are now available with a fabric chest strap that is considerably more comfortable than the plastic ones.)

Start monitoring. Once you know how to wear your monitor and get a reading, and you have a feel for the button(s), you're ready to begin working out with it. In your first few workouts with the monitor I suggest that you put it on, do your normal workout, and look at the display every few minutes without yet worrying about your target heart rate or any other function. Simply get used to working out with one.

Program your zones. Two or three such workouts should have you ready to transform your new heart rate monitor from a toy into a tool. A heart rate monitor becomes a tool when you actively use it to control your level of effort in workouts. This is where target heart rate zones come in.

The number of programmable heart rate zones varies by model. Some units have just one target zone that you can change from one workout to the next. Others have three zones, and still others offer five. In addition, some monitors use automatically programmed zones, while others allow you to program them manually.

In order to use a heart rate monitor effectively with your Lean Look cardio workouts, the device must allow you to program your target zones manually. Here's how to go about it. Wear your monitor while performing a Lean Look cardio workout as prescribed. As you near completion of your last interval, note your heart rate. It's important that you use the plus-one rule correctly, so that you complete the last interval at the same level of effort at which you started the first interval and feel that you could complete one and only more interval at the same level of effort before reaching total exhaustion. If this is the case, then the heart rate number you see at the end of your last interval represents the top of the target heart rate zone. To establish the bottom limit of the target zone, subtract 10 beats per minute from the maximum.

For example, let's say you are doing a long interval workout with four 4-minute intervals. At the end of the fourth interval your heart rate is 167 BPM (beats per minute). This number represents the upper limit of your target heart rate zone for 4-minute intervals. Now subtract 10 BPM from 167 BPM, which yields 157 BPM. This number represents the lower limit of your target heart rate zone for 4-minute intervals. Next, consult the owner's manual for your heart rate monitor and figure out how to program this zone (157 to 167 BPM) into the device. Once you've done this you can use the device to ensure that you are working at the appropriate intensity in each of your subsequent 4-minute interval workouts.

You probably won't find heart rate monitoring very useful when doing very short intervals—namely, 20-second power intervals and 30-second speed intervals—because of a phenomenon known as *cardiac lag*. When you suddenly increase the intensity of exercise from a low, warm-up, or active recovery intensity to a very high intensity, it takes some time for your heart rate to plateau at that particular intensity level. In very short intervals, your hard effort will be all but over by the time your heart rate reaches this level, so your heart rate monitor will not be very useful for controlling effort intensity in this circumstance.

Cardiac lag is not a problem in longer intervals (intervals over 1 minute), and in fact it is already accounted for in the target zones. Your heart rate should climb up to the lower limit of your target zone within 30 seconds of your beginning an interval. It should continue to climb toward the top of the zone, without exceeding the upper limit, and without any increase in your effort level as you continue through the interval. If your heart rate does this, you know you're doing the interval at the right effort level.

Expect your target heart rate zones to change over time. As you gain fitness, the heart rate associated with any given level of effort will decrease. You will also find that sustaining any given heart rate feels easier and easier, and that you can sustain higher heart rates longer before feeling fatigued. For example, suppose you do your cardio workouts on a stationary bike that allows you to see how many watts of power you are generating at any given time. (Power happens to be a direct measurement of exercise effort output.) Let's say that when you first begin doing 4-minute intervals using the target heart rate zone of 157–167 BPM from our previous example, you find yourself producing approximately 160 watts. After a few weeks of consistent training, you might find yourself producing 170 watts at the same heart rate, and yet it feels easier. This means you've gotten fitter and it's time to readjust your target heart rate zone for 4-minute intervals.

How do you do this? Simply repeat the process you used to establish the initial zone. You might find that your upper limit is now 170 BPM, making your new target heart rate zone for four-minute intervals 160–170 BPM. You might also note that your average watts are a little higher—perhaps 175—at this heart rate.

When working with some of my over-motivated clients (who are usually competitive athletes), I prescribe heart rate monitor training primarily as a means to keep them from working too hard. A typical case was J.D., a college hockey player I worked with. J.D. was a workaholic who trained too hard for his own good. When I started working with him, he was following a summer workout created by his team's strength coach. The issue was that he was adding exercises, increasing intensities, and not taking his scheduled days off.

I explained to J.D. why a heart rate monitor was important to him, and then I showed him how to use it to assess the proper intensity for each workout; to gauge when he was working too hard; and even to determine when he was not fully recovered from previous workouts and becoming "overtrained." By giving him tangible numbers that he could understand, I made J.D. an instant believer in his training program.

PHASE III

Commit your results to memory. Virtually all monitors have a memory feature that allows you to store information (workout duration, average heart rate, time in target zone, calories burned, etc.) from one or more workouts for later review. The most basic monitors store just one workout, so if you want to record the numbers in a written exercise log, you must do so before you use the monitor again. Some of the more expensive monitors allow you to store literally hundreds of workouts and download them to your personal computer. As is the case with body fat measurements, workout information keeps you motivated when you can see numerical proof that you're getting fitter.

Learn your monitor's advanced functions and features. While individual heart rate monitors function differently from one to another, the one function they all share is real-time display of your current heart rate. Some models provide this readout automatically as soon as you put on the chest strap. With others—namely those that have a stopwatch function—you may have to enter the "monitor" or "chrono" mode to display your heart rate. Note that your workout does not necessarily begin as soon as you have a heart rate readout. All models require that you press a button to begin a formal, timed workout. In a basic, one-button monitor there is no readout of elapsed workout time.

In models that have a stopwatch you must start the stopwatch (or timer) to begin a formal workout. The heart rate monitors that offer the most workout information are those that are integrated with speed and distance devices for runners and those that are integrated with bike computers for cyclists. With the latter you can observe not only your heart rate and workout time but also your speed, power output, pedaling cadence, average speed, and other data—not necessarily all at once, but by flipping modes as you continue pedaling.

Another bit of information you might want to track during workouts is calories burned. This requires a heart rate monitor that has a feature that counts calories burned during a workout based on your weight and heart rate. Other features available in higher-end models expand the range of what you can do with your heart rate monitor. I hope this overview will help you choose the monitor that is best for you and get the most out of it.

IT'S ABOUT FEEDBACK

It would be difficult to overstate the importance of feedback to an effective exercise program, including the Lean Look program. The right kind of feedback information can be highly motivating and helps take some of the guesswork out of training. A heart rate monitor is one of the best exercise feedback devices you can use. But it can't motivate you or take the guesswork out of your training unless you learn how to use it properly. So, if you choose to use a heart rate monitor, take the step-by-step approach outlined here and you'll be in the zone in no time!

CHAPTER 16

Lean for Life

Becoming substantially leaner over the course of 12 weeks, as you will do in this program, is a significant accomplishment, but you don't want to stop there. The larger goal is to make continued progress until you achieve your true optimal body composition, and then to maintain it for life. In this chapter I will show you how to achieve this larger goal by transforming the basic structure of the Lean Look program into a year-round cycle that you can repeat indefinitely.

Once again, competitive athletes provide an example to follow. The competitive athletes I work with train in annual "periodization cycles," which ensure that they keep moving forward throughout the year and from one year to the next. Training in this way also prevents boredom. Each sport has its own approach to periodization. The approach I recommend for noncompetitive athletes like you borrows a little from strength sports such as football and a little from endurance sports such as running.

There's something magical about training in yearlong cycles. Part of the magic lies in the fact that when you use these cycles, your training is continually changing—not randomly, but in a consistent direction—so that you're always stimulating new progress in your body. Part of the magic also lies in the fact that with periodization cycles you don't commit the same amount of time and energy to exercise every week throughout the year. Instead you start with a smaller investment and gradually build throughout the year until you reach a fitness peak; then you take a little break and start over again. Granted, when you near that peak you are training harder than you would want to train consistently over a long period of time. But overall, when you look at the cycle as a whole, you can actually get better results from a smaller total investment of time and energy.

I create yearlong training plans for many of my clients who understand the benefits of taking the long view. One example that comes to mind is that of Eric, a thirty-nine-year-old father, salesman, and student who had been recently diagnosed with type 2 diabetes with elevated cholesterol when he called me up seeking help. Eric's wife was a big factor in helping him eat better. She was a great cook who enthusiastically prepared meals according to his doctor's recommendations. But in looking at Eric's lifestyle I could see that the exercise component was going to be a challenge. He had no free time—period! His two-year-old son, work, and school commitments completely filled his days, including weekends.

My initial visit with Eric was at his home with his wife. As soon as I walked in I saw that his dog (a Labrador retriever) was overweight. A good friend once told me that if your dog is overweight, you don't exercise enough! So I suggested that henceforward family time every day include walking the dog. Each week their walk time increased. I also added exercises in which Eric held his son and performed movements at his home and while walking.

I set up a 52-week training program and progress chart for Eric and his wife. I had them both purchase pedometers and heart rate monitors to track their activity better. The program included heart rate intensities, step distances on the pedometers, rest days, easy days and tough days. This structure helped Eric plan his days and weeks much more efficiently and healthfully.

I get frequent updates from the couple. They still walk and on some days they jog with a baby jogger. Eric has lost 21 pounds and feels great. His blood sugar has been under control for 18 months and his cholesterol has significantly decreased, although it still needs to be lower. We're working on that. And the dog is fit and acts like a puppy.

The one-year plan I will give you here is a little different, but it should be even more effective. As you know, the 12-week Lean Look program presented in this book has three phases. Your annual Lean Look periodization cycle will have four phases that line up with the seasons: winter, spring, summer, and fall. Each phase is 12 weeks long. This leaves four weeks of the year unaccounted for. You can dispose of these four weeks however you see fit. You can take a 1-week break after each season, spend four weeks in the winter participating in other types of fitness activities that are not a part of your normal routine, or do whatever you think is best for you.

The winter is a base building period in which you focus on developing a new foundation of aerobic fitness and muscle balance. In the spring it's time to pump up the intensity with challenging strength-building workouts and short cardio intervals. In the summer, shift your focus toward power development and intermediate intervals. In the fall, put an emphasis on building muscular and cardiovascular endurance.

There are three new types of cardio workout and one new type of strength workout that you will incorporate into the annual Lean Look periodization cycle. The first new cardio workout is a non-interval workout that I call a *foundation workout*. It consists of a sustained, steady effort of moderate intensity that serves to build cardio fitness and endurance. Although, as I've stated, high-intensity cardio intervals are more efficient fat-burning workouts, foundation workouts have their place, too. Because you can sustain a moderate effort level longer than a high effort level, you can burn more total fat in foundation workouts by increasing their duration beyond what is possible in interval workouts.

The second new type of cardio workout is called a *tempo workout*. It consists of a single, sustained effort of 10 to 20 minutes at a moderately high intensity sandwiched between a 5-minute warm-up and a 5-minute cooldown. *The plus-one rule does not apply to tempo workouts.* Instead use a plus-five standard to guide your effort. Do the tempo portion of your tempo workouts at the highest work level you feel you could sustain 5 minutes longer than the workout requires you to do. For example, if the workout calls for a 10-minute tempo interval, do it at an effort level you feel you could sustain for 15 minutes and no longer.

The third new type of cardio workout is a *mixed intervals workout.* As the name implies, this type of workout combines intervals of various durations ranging between 1 minute and 6 minutes. In these workouts 1-minute intervals are followed by 2-minute active recoveries, 2-minute and 3-minute intervals are followed by 3-minute active recoveries, and 4-minute intervals are followed by 4-minute active recoveries. A 6-minute interval is always the last in a mixed interval workout and is therefore followed immediately by a 5-minute cooldown.

There is also one new type of strength workout that you will incorporate into your annual Lean Look periodization cycle—a "muscular endurance workout." Like the workouts you did in the three phases of the 12-week Lean Look program, this workout uses a circuit format, and it also uses the same exercises that are appropriate for strength-building workouts. The only difference is that you do more repetitions of each exercise—shoot for 15—using a lighter weight. For example, if you choose to include the Squat with Dumbbells (see page 151) in a muscular endurance resistance workout, use a lighter set of dumbbells than you do in the strength-building version of this exercise and increase the number of repetitions you complete from 12 to 15. Use the plus-one rule to select the appropriate weight for each exercise in a muscular endurance workout.

The following charts provide an example of a yearlong Lean Look periodization cycle. You can adjust the challenge level of the workouts as appropriate.

WINTER TRAINING EMPHASES: MUSCLE BALANCE AND CARDIO FOUNDATION

Wk #	Sunday	Monday	Tuesday	Wednesday	Thursday	Friday	Saturday
1	Rest	Muscle-Balancing 1 set 6 exercises	Cardio Foundation 20 minutes	Muscle-Balancing 1 set 6 exercises	Cardio Foundation 20 minutes	Muscle-Balancing 1 set 6 exercises	Cardio Foundation 20 minutes
2	Rest	Muscle-Balancing 1 set 9 exercises	Cardio Foundation 22 minutes	Muscle-Balancing 1 set 6 exercises	Cardio Foundation 22 minutes	Muscle-Balancing 1 set 6 exercises	Cardio Foundation 22 minutes
3	Rest	Muscle-Balancing 1 set 6 exercises	Cardio Power Intervals 6 X 20 seconds	Muscle-Balancing 1 set 6 exercises	Cardio Foundation 24 minutes	Muscle-Balancing 1 set 6 exercises	Cardio Foundation 24 minutes
4	Rest	Muscle-Balancing 1 set 6 exercises	Cardio Power Intervals 6 X 20 seconds	Muscle-Balancing 1 set 6 exercises	Cardio Foundation 20 minutes	Muscle-Balancing 1 set 6 exercises	Cardio Foundation 20 minutes
5	Rest	Muscle-Balancing 1 set 9 exercises	Cardio Power Intervals 8 X 20 seconds	Muscle-Balancing 1 set 9 exercises	Cardio Foundation 26 minutes	Muscle-Balancing 1 set 9 exercises	Cardio Foundation 26 minutes
6	Rest	Muscle-Balancing 2 sets 9 exercises	Cardio Power Intervals 10 X 20 seconds	Muscle-Balancing 1 set 9 exercises	Cardio Foundation 28 minutes	Muscle-Balancing 1 set 9 exercises	Cardio Foundation 28 minutes
7	Rest	Muscle-Balancing 2 sets 9 exercises	Cardio Power Intervals 12 X 20 seconds	Muscle-Balancing 2 sets 9 exercises	Cardio Speed Intervals 4 X 1 minute	Muscle-Balancing 2 sets 9 exercises	Cardio Foundation 30 minutes
8	Rest	Muscle-Balancing 1 set 9 exercises	Cardio Power Intervals 6 X 20 seconds	Muscle-Balancing 1 set 9 exercises	Cardio Speed Intervals 4 X 1 minute	Muscle-Balancing 1 set 9 exercises	Cardio Foundation 24 minutes
9	Rest	Muscle-Balancing 2 sets 9 exercises	Cardio Speed Intervals 6 X 30 seconds	Muscle-Balancing 2 sets 9 exercises	Cardio Speed Intervals 5 X 1 minute	Muscle-Balancing 2 sets 9 exercises	Cardio Foundation 30 minutes
10	Rest	Muscle-Balancing 2 sets 12 exercises	Cardio Speed Intervals 8 X 30 seconds	Muscle-Balancing 2 sets 9 exercises	Cardio Speed Intervals 6 X 1 minute	Muscle-Balancing 2 sets 9 exercises	Cardio Foundation 32 minutes
11	Rest	Muscle-Balancing 2 sets 12 exercises	Cardio Speed Intervals 10 X 30 seconds	Muscle-Balancing 2 sets 12 exercises	Cardio Speed Intervals 7 X 1 minute	Muscle-Balancing 2 sets 12 exercises	Cardio Foundation 34 minutes
12	Rest	Muscle-Balancing 2 sets 9 exercises	Cardio Speed Intervals 6 X 30 seconds	Muscle-Balancing 2 sets 9 exercises	Cardio Speed Intervals 5 X 1 minute	Muscle-Balancing 2 sets 9 exercises	Cardio Foundation 28 minutes

SPRING TRAINING EMPHASES: STRENGTH BUILDING AND AEROBIC CAPACITY

Wk #	Sunday	Monday	Tuesday	Wednesday	Thursday	Friday	Saturday
1	Rest	Strength - Building 1 set 9 exercises	Cardio Intervals 3 X 2 minutes	Muscle-Balancing 2 sets 12 exercises	Cardio Speed Intervals 6 X 1 minute	Strength - Building 1 set 9 exercises	Cardio Foundation 30 minutes
2	Rest	Strength - Building 2 sets 9 exercises	Cardio Intervals 4 X 2 minutes	Muscle-Balancing 2 sets 12 exercises	Cardio Speed Intervals 7 X 1 minute	Strength - Building 2 sets 9 exercises	Cardio Foundation 32 minutes
3	Rest	Strength - Building 2 sets 9 exercises	Cardio Intervals 4 X 2 minutes	Muscle-Balancing 3 sets 12 exercises	Cardio Speed Intervals 8 X 1 minute	Strength - Building 2 sets 9 exercises	Cardio Foundation 34 minutes
4	Rest	Strength - Building 1 set 9 exercises	Cardio Intervals 3 X 2 minutes	Muscle-Balancing 2 sets 12 exercises	Cardio Speed Intervals 6 X 1 minute	Strength - Building 1 set 9 exercises	Cardio Foundation 30 minutes
5	Rest	Strength - Building 2 sets 9 exercises	Cardio Intervals 4 X 2 minutes	Muscle-Balancing 3 sets 12 exercises	Cardio Int. Intervals 2 X 3 minutes	Strength - Building 2 sets 9 exercises	Cardio Foundation 32 minutes
6	Rest	Strength - Building 2 sets 12 exercises	Cardio Intervals 5 X 2 minutes	Muscle-Balancing 3 sets 12 exercises	Cardio Int. Intervals 2 X 3 minutes	Strength - Building 2 sets 12 exercises	Cardio Foundation 34 minutes
7	Rest	Strength - Building 2 sets 12 exercises	Cardio Intervals 5 X 2 minutes	Muscle-Balancing 3 sets 12 exercises	Cardio Int. Intervals 3 X 3 minutes	Strength - Building 2 sets 12 exercises	Cardio Foundation 36 minutes
8	Rest	Strength - Building 2 sets 9 exercises	Cardio Intervals 4 X 2 minutes	Muscle-Balancing 1 set 9 exercises	Cardio Int. Intervals 2 X 3 minutes	Strength - Building 2 sets 9 exercises	Cardio Foundation 32 minutes
9	Rest	Strength - Building 2 sets 12 exercises	Cardio Intervals 5 X 2 minutes	Muscle-Balancing 2 sets 12 exercises	Cardio Int. Intervals 3 X 3 minutes	Strength - Building 2 sets 12 exercises	Cardio Foundation 34 minutes
10	Rest	Strength - Building 3 sets 12 exercises	Cardio Intervals 5 X 2 minutes	Muscle-Balancing 2 sets 9 exercises	Cardio Int. Intervals 4 X 3 minutes	Strength - Building 3 sets 12 exercises	Cardio Foundation 36 minutes
11	Rest	Strength - Building 3 sets 12 exercises	Cardio Intervals 6 X 2 minutes	Muscle-Balancing 2 sets 9 exercises	Cardio Int. Intervals 4 X 3 minutes	Strength - Building 3 sets 12 exercises	Cardio Foundation 38 minutes
12	Rest	Strength - Building 2 sets 9 exercises	Cardio Intervals 4 X 2 minutes	Muscle-Balancing 2 sets 12 exercises	Cardio Int. Intervals 3 X 3 minutes	Strength - Building 2 sets 9 exercises	Cardio Foundation 30 minutes

SUMMER TRAINING EMPHASES: MUSCLE POWER AND INTENSIVE ENDURANCE

Wk #	Sunday	Monday	Tuesday	Wednesday	Thursday	Friday	Saturday
1	Rest	Power 1 set 9 exercises	Cardio Tempo 10 min. hard 20 min. total	Strength-Building 2 sets 9 exercises	Cardio Mixed Intervals 1 min. interval 6 min. interval	Strength-Building 2 sets 9 exercises	Cardio Foundation 32 minutes
2	Rest	Power 2 sets 9 exercises	Cardio Tempo 12 min. hard 22 min. total	Strength-Building 3 sets 9 exercisess	Cardio Mixed Intervals 1-3-6	Strength-Building 3 sets 9 exercises	Cardio Foundation 34 minutes
3	Rest	Power 2 sets 9 exercises	Cardio Tempo 14 min. hard 24 min. total	Strength-Building 3 sets 12 exercises	Cardio Mixed Intervals 1-3-6	Strength-Building 3 sets 9 exercises	Cardio Foundation 36 minutes
4	Rest	Power 1 set 9 exercises	Cardio Tempo 10 min. hard 20 min. total	Strength-Building 2 sets 9 exercises	Cardio Mixed Intervals 1-6l	Strength-Building 2 sets 9 exercises	Cardio Foundation 32 minutes
5	Rest	Power 2 sets 9 exercises	Cardio Tempo 14 min. hard 24 min. total	Strength-Building 3 sets 9 exercises	Cardio Mixed Intervals 1-3-6	Power 2 sets 9 exercises	Cardio Foundation 34 minutes
6	Rest	Power 2 sets 12 exercises	Cardio Tempo 16 min. hard 26 min. total	Strength-Building 3 sets 9 exercises	Cardio Mixed Intervals 1-2-3-6	Power 2 sets 12 exercisess	Cardio Foundation 36 minutes
7	Rest	Power 2 sets 12 exercises	Cardio Tempo 18 min. hard 28 min. totals	Strength-Building 3 sets 9 exercises	Cardio Mixed Intervals 1-2-3-6	Power 2 sets 12 exercises	Cardio Foundation 38 minutes
8	Rest	Power 2 sets 9 exercises	Cardio Tempo 14 min. hard 24 min. total	Strength-Building 2 sets 9 exercises	Cardio Mixed Intervals 1-3-6	Power 2 sets 9 exercises	Cardio Foundation 32 minutes
9	Rest	Power 2 sets 12 exercises	Cardio Tempo 18 min. hard 28 min. total	Strength-Building 3 sets 9 exercises	Cardio Mixed Intervals 1-2-3-6	Power 2 sets 12 exercises	Cardio Foundation 36 minutes
10	Rest	Power 3 sets 12 exercises	Cardio Tempo 20 min. hard 30 min. total	Strength-Building 3 sets 9 exercises	Cardio Mixed Intervals 1-2-3-4-6	Power 3 sets 12 exercises	Cardio Foundation 38 minutes
11	Rest	Power 2 sets 12 exercises	Cardio Tempo 20 min. hard 30 min. total	Strength-Building 3 sets 9 exercises	Cardio Mixed Intervals 1-2-3-4-6	Power 2 sets 12 exercises	Cardio Foundation 40 minutes
12	Rest	Power 2 sets 9 exercises	Cardio Tempo 14 min. hard 24 min. total	Strength-Building 2 sets 9 exercises	Cardio Mixed Intervals 1-2-3-6	Power 2 sets 9 exercises	Cardio Foundation 32 minutes

FALL TRAINING EMPHASES: MUSCULAR ENDURANCE AND CARDIOVASCULAR ENDURANCE

Wk #	Sunday	Monday	Tuesday	Wednesday	Thursday	Friday	Saturday
1	Rest	Muscular endurance 2 sets 9 exercises	Cardio Foundation 32 minutes	Power 2 sets 9 exercises	Cardio Tempo 18 min. hard 28 min. total	Muscular endurance 2 sets 9 exercises	Cardio Foundation 36 minutes
2	Rest	Muscular endurance 2 sets 12 exercises	Cardio Foundation 34 minutes	Strength-Building 3 sets 9 exercises	Cardio Tempo 20 min. hard 30 min. total	Muscular endurance 2 sets 12 exercises	Cardio Foundation 38 minutes
3	Rest	Muscular endurance 2 sets 12 exercises	Cardio Foundation 36 minutes	Muscle-Balancing 3 sets 9 exercises	Cardio Tempo 22 min. hard 32 min. total	Muscular endurance 2 sets 12 exercises	Cardio Foundation 40 minutes
4	Rest	Muscular endurance 2 sets 9 exercises	Cardio Foundation 32 minutes	Power 2 sets 9 exercises	Cardio Tempo 14 min. hard 24 min. total	Muscular endurance 2 sets 9 exercises	Cardio Foundation 32 minutes
5	Rest	Muscular endurance 2 sets 12 exercises	Cardio Foundation 34 minutes	Strength-Building 3 sets 9 exercises	Cardio Tempo 20 min. hard 30 min. total	Muscular endurance 2 sets 12 exercises	Cardio Foundation 38 minutes
6	Rest	Muscular endurance 3 sets 12 exercises	Cardio Foundation 36 minutes	Muscle Balancing 3 sets 9 exercises	Cardio Tempo 22 min. hard 32 min. total	Muscular endurance 3 sets 12 exercises	Cardio Foundation 40 minutes
7	Rest	Muscular endurance 3 sets 12 exercises	Cardio Foundation 38 minutes	Power 3 sets 9 exercises	Cardio Tempo 24 min. hard 34 min. total	Muscular endurance 3 sets 12 exercises	Cardio Foundation 42 minutes
8	Rest	Muscular endurance 2 sets 12 exercises	Cardio Foundation 32 minutes	Strength-Building 2 sets 9 exercises	Cardio Tempo 16 min. hard 26 min. total	Muscular endurance 2 sets 12 exercises	Cardio Foundation 36 minutes
9	Rest	Muscular endurance 3 sets 12 exercises	Cardio Foundation 36 minutes	Muscle-Balancing 3 sets 9 exercises	Cardio Tempo 22 min. hard 32 min. total	Muscular endurance 3 sets 12 exercises	Cardio Foundation 42 minutes
10	Rest	Muscular endurance 3 sets 12 exercises	Cardio Foundation 38 minutes	Power 3 sets 9 exercises	Cardio Tempo 24 min. hard 34 min. total	Muscular endurance 3 sets 12 exercises	Cardio Foundation 44 minutes
11	Rest	Muscular endurance 3 sets 12 exercises	Cardio Foundation 40 minutes	Strength-Building 3 sets 9 exercises	Cardio Tempo 26 min. hard 36 min. total	Muscular endurance 3 sets 12 exercises	Cardio Foundation 46 minutes
12	Rest	Muscular endurance 2 sets 9 exercises	Cardio Foundation 32 minutes	Muscle-Balancing 2 sets 9 exercises	Cardio Tempo 18 min. hard 28 min. total	Muscular endurance 2 sets 9 exercises	Cardio Foundation 36 minutes

WHAT ABOUT NUTRITION?

As for nutrition, the guidelines provided for the nutrition component of the three phases of the Lean Look program will last you a lifetime. If you have not fully implemented all 10 of the key substitutions presented in Phase I by the end of the 12-week program and you still have excess body fat to lose, keep making substitutions until you have fully implemented all of them. The same advice applies to the eight nutrient timing practices of Phase II. And there is no deadline for making the decision to experiment with any of the supplements I introduced to you in Phase III. By tying up these nutritional "loose ends" while following the annual Lean Look periodization plan detailed in this chapter, you will take that final step toward achieving the leanest, healthiest body you can achieve.

APPENDIX A

Body Fat Estimation Tables for Use with the Tape Measure Method

I n this appendix you will find percent body fat estimation tables based on a formula developed by the U.S. Navy, which relies on body circumference measurements. To use these tables you must generate a circumference value using the tape measure method discussed in chapter 2. You must also know your height in inches. The tables are organized by gender and height. Be sure to use the correct table!

MEN'S TABLES

PERCENT BODY FAT ESTIMATION FOR MEN (HEIGHT RANGE 5'0" to 5'4½")

CIRCUMFERENCE VALUE	HEIGHT IN INCHES									
	60.0	60.5	61.0	61.5	62.0	62.5	63.0	63.5	64.0	64.5
13.5	9	9								
14.0	11	11	10	10	10	10	9	9		
14.5	12	12	12	11	11	11	11	10	10	10
15.0	13	13	13	13	12	12	12	12	11	11
15.5	15	14	14	14	14	13	13	13	13	12
16.0	16	16	15	15	15	15	14	14	14	14
16.5	17	17	16	16	16	16	15	15	15	15
17.0	18	18	18	17	17	17	17	16	16	16
17.5	19	19	19	18	18	18	18	17	17	17
18.0	20	20	20	19	19	19	19	18	18	18
18.5	21	21	21	20	20	20	20	19	19	19
19.0	22	22	22	21	21	21	21	20	20	20
19.5	23	23	23	22	22	22	22	21	21	21
20.0	24	24	24	23	23	23	23	22	22	22
20.5	25	25	25	24	24	24	24	23	23	23
21.0	26	26	25	25	25	25	24	24	24	24
21.5	27	27	26	26	26	26	25	25	25	25
22.0	28	27	27	27	27	26	26	26	26	25
22.5	29	28	28	28	28	27	27	27	27	26
23.0	29	29	29	29	28	28	28	28	27	27
23.5	30	30	30	29	29	29	29	28	28	28
24.0	31	31	30	30	30	30	29	29	29	29
24.5	32	31	31	31	31	30	30	30	30	29
25.0	32	32	32	32	31	31	31	31	30	30
25.5	33	33	33	32	32	32	32	31	31	31
26.0	34	34	33	33	33	33	32	32	32	32
26.5	35	34	34	34	34	33	33	33	33	32
27.0	35	35	35	35	34	34	34	34	33	33
27.5	36	36	36	35	35	35	35	34	34	34

28.0	37	36	36	36	36	35	35	35	35	34
28.5			37	37	36	36	36	36	35	35
29.0					37	37	37	36	36	36
29.5								37	37	36

PERCENT BODY FAT ESTIMATION FOR MEN (HEIGHT RANGE 5'5" to 5'9½")

CIRCUMFERENCE VALUE	HEIGHT IN INCHES									
	65.0	65.5	66.0	66.5	67.0	67.5	68.0	68.5	69.0	69.5
14.5	10	9	9							
15.0	11	11	10	10	10	10	10	9	9	
15.5	12	12	12	11	11	11	11	11	10	10
16.0	13	13	13	13	12	12	12	12	12	11
16.5	14	14	14	14	14	13	13	13	13	12
17.0	16	15	15	15	15	14	14	14	14	14
17.5	17	16	16	16	16	16	15	15	15	15
18.0	18	18	17	17	17	17	16	16	16	16
18.5	19	19	18	18	18	18	17	17	17	17
19.0	20	20	19	19	19	19	18	18	18	18
19.5	21	21	20	20	20	20	19	19	19	19
20.0	22	21	21	21	21	21	20	20	20	20
20.5	23	22	22	22	22	21	21	21	21	21
21.0	24	23	23	23	23	22	22	22	22	21
21.5	24	24	24	24	23	23	23	23	23	22
22.0	25	25	25	25	24	24	24	24	23	23
22.5	26	26	26	25	25	25	25	24	24	24
23.0	27	27	26	26	26	26	26	25	25	25
23.5	28	27	27	27	27	27	26	26	26	26
24.0	28	28	28	28	28	27	27	27	27	26
24.5	29	29	29	29	28	28	28	28	27	27
25.0	30	30	30	29	29	29	29	28	28	28
25.5	31	31	30	30	30	30	29	29	29	29
26.0	31	31	31	31	31	30	30	30	30	29
26.5	32	32	32	32	31	31	31	31	30	30
27.0	33	33	32	32	32	32	32	31	31	31
27.5	34	33	33	33	33	32	32	32	32	32
28.0	34	34	34	34	33	33	33	33	32	32

28.5	35	35	34	34	34	34	34	33	33	33
29.0	36	35	35	35	35	34	34	34	34	34
29.5	36	36	36	36	35	35	35	35	34	34
30.0	37	37	36	36	36	36	35	35	35	35
30.5			37	37	37	36	36	36	36	35
31.0						37	37	36	36	36
31.5									37	37

PERCENT BODY FAT ESTIMATION FOR MEN (HEIGHT RANGE 5'10" to 6'2½")

CIRCUMFERENCE VALUE	HEIGHT IN INCHES									
	70.0	70.5	71.0	71.5	72.0	72.5	73.0	73.5	74.0	74.5
15.5	10	10	9	9	9					
16.0	11	11	11	10	10	10	10	10	9	9
16.5	12	12	12	12	11	11	11	11	11	10
17.0	13	13	13	13	13	12	12	12	12	11
17.5	14	14	14	14	14	13	13	13	13	13
18.0	15	15	15	15	15	14	14	14	14	14
18.5	17	16	16	16	16	15	15	15	15	15
19.0	18	17	17	17	17	16	16	16	16	16
19.5	18	18	18	18	18	17	17	17	17	17
20.0	19	19	19	19	19	18	18	18	18	18
20.5	20	20	20	20	19	19	19	19	19	18
21.0	21	21	21	21	20	20	20	20	20	19
21.5	22	22	22	21	21	21	21	21	20	20
22.0	23	23	23	22	22	22	22	22	21	21
22.5	24	24	23	23	23	23	23	22	22	22
23.0	25	24	24	24	24	24	23	23	23	23
23.5	25	25	25	25	25	24	24	24	24	24
24.0	26	26	26	26	25	25	25	25	25	24
24.5	27	27	27	26	26	26	26	26	25	25
25.0	28	28	27	27	27	27	26	26	26	26
25.5	29	28	28	28	28	27	27	27	27	27
26.0	29	29	29	29	28	28	28	28	28	27
26.5	30	30	30	29	29	29	29	28	28	28
27.0	31	30	30	30	30	30	29	29	29	29
27.5	31	31	31	31	30	30	30	30	30	29

28.0	32	32	32	31	31	31	31	31	30	30
28.5	33	32	32	32	32	32	31	31	31	31
29.0	33	33	33	33	32	32	32	32	32	31
29.5	34	34	34	33	33	33	33	32	32	32
30.0	35	34	34	34	34	34	33	33	33	33
30.5	35	35	35	35	34	34	34	34	34	33
31.0	36	36	35	35	35	35	35	34	34	34
31.5	36	36	36	36	36	35	35	35	35	35
32.0	37	37	37	36	36	36	36	36	35	35
32.5				37	37	36	36	36	36	36
33.0							37	37	36	36
33.5										37

PERCENT BODY FAT ESTIMATION FOR MEN (HEIGHT RANGE 6'3" to 6'7½")

CIRCUMFERENCE VALUE	HEIGHT IN INCHES									
	75.0	75.5	76.0	76.5	77.0	77.5	78.0	78.5	79.0	79.5
16.5	10	10	10	10	9	9				
17.0	11	11	11	11	10	10	10	10	10	9
17.5	12	12	12	12	12	11	11	11	11	11
18.0	13	13	13	13	13	12	12	12	12	12
18.5	14	14	14	14	14	13	13	13	13	13
19.0	15	15	15	15	15	14	14	14	14	14
19.5	16	16	16	16	16	15	15	15	15	15
20.0	17	17	17	17	17	16	16	16	16	16
20.5	18	18	18	18	17	17	17	17	17	16
21.0	19	19	19	19	18	18	18	18	18	17
21.5	20	20	20	19	19	19	19	19	18	18
22.0	21	21	20	20	20	20	20	20	19	19
22.5	22	22	21	21	21	21	21	20	20	20
23.0	23	22	22	22	22	22	21	21	21	21
23.5	23	23	23	23	23	22	22	22	22	22
24.0	24	24	24	24	23	23	23	23	23	22
24.5	25	25	25	24	24	24	24	24	23	23
25.0	26	25	25	25	25	25	24	24	24	24
25.5	26	26	26	26	26	25	25	25	25	25
26.0	27	27	27	27	26	26	26	26	26	25

26.5	28	28	27	27	27	27	27	26	26	26
27.0	29	28	28	28	28	28	27	27	27	27
27.5	29	29	29	29	28	28	28	28	28	27
28.0	30	30	29	29	29	29	29	29	28	28
28.5	31	30	30	30	30	30	29	29	29	29
29.0	31	31	31	31	30	30	30	30	30	29
29.5	32	32	31	31	31	31	31	30	30	30
30.0	32	32	32	32	32	31	31	31	31	31
30.5	33	33	33	32	32	32	32	32	32	31
31.0	34	33	33	33	33	33	33	32	32	32
31.5	34	34	34	34	33	33	33	33	33	33
32.0	35	35	34	34	34	34	34	33	33	33
32.5	35	35	35	35	35	34	34	34	34	34
33.0	36	36	36	35	35	35	35	35	34	34
33.5	37	36	36	36	36	36	35	35	35	35
34.0		37	37	37	36	36	36	36	36	35
34.5					37	37	37	36	36	36
35.0								37	37	36

WOMEN'S TABLES

PERCENT BODY FAT ESTIMATION FOR WOMEN (HEIGHT RANGE 4'10" to 5'2½")

CIRCUMFERENCE VALUE	HEIGHT IN INCHES									
	58.0	59.5	59.0	59.5	60.0	60.5	61.0	61.5	62.0	62.5
45.0	19									
45.5	20	20	19							
46.0	21	20	20	20	19					
46.5	21	21	21	20	20	20	19	19		
47.0	22	22	22	21	21	20	20	20	19	19
47.5	23	23	22	22	22	21	21	21	20	20
48.0	24	23	23	23	22	22	22	21	21	21
48.5	24	24	24	23	23	23	22	22	22	21
49.0	25	25	24	24	24	23	23	23	22	22
49.5	26	26	25	25	24	24	24	23	23	23
50.0	27	26	26	26	25	25	24	24	24	23
50.5	27	27	27	26	26	26	25	25	25	24
51.0	28	28	27	27	27	26	26	26	25	25
51.5	29	28	28	28	27	27	27	26	26	26
52.0	29	29	29	28	28	28	27	27	27	26
52.5	30	30	29	29	29	28	28	28	27	27
53.0	31	30	30	30	29	29	29	28	28	28
53.5	31	31	31	30	30	30	29	29	29	28
54.0	32	32	31	31	31	30	30	30	29	29
54.5	33	32	32	32	31	31	31	30	30	30
55.0	33	33	33	32	32	32	31	31	31	30
55.5	34	34	33	33	33	32	32	32	31	31
56.0	35	34	34	34	33	33	33	32	32	31
56.5	35	35	35	34	34	34	33	33	32	32
57.0	36	36	35	35	34	34	34	33	33	33
57.5	37	36	36	35	35	35	34	34	34	33
58.0	37	37	36	36	36	35	35	35	34	34
58.5	38	37	37	37	36	36	36	35	35	35
59.0	38	38	38	37	37	37	36	36	36	35

59.5	39	39	38	38	38	37	37	36	36	36
60.0	40	39	39	38	38	38	37	37	37	36
60.5	40	40	39	39	39	38	38	38	37	37
61.0	41	40	40	40	39	39	39	38	38	38
61.5	41	41	41	40	40	40	39	39	38	38
62.0	42	42	41	41	40	40	40	39	39	39
62.5	42	42	42	41	41	41	40	40	40	39
63.0	43	43	42	42	42	41	41	41	40	40
63.5	44	43	43	42	42	42	41	41	41	40
64.0	44	44	43	43	43	42	42	42	41	41
64.5	45	44	44	44	43	43	43	42	42	42
65.0	45	45	45	44	44	43	43	43	42	42
65.5	46	45	45	45	44	44	44	43	43	43
66.0	46	46	46	45	45	45	44	44	43	43
66.5	47	46	46	46	45	45	45	44	44	44
67.0			47	46	46	46	45	45	45	44
67.5				47	46	46	46	45	45	45
68.0					47	47	46	46	46	45
68.5							47	46	46	46
69.0								47	47	46
69.5										47

PERCENT BODY FAT ESTIMATION FOR WOMEN (HEIGHT RANGE 5'3" to 5'7½")

CIRCUMFERENCE VALUE	HEIGHT IN INCHES									
	63.0	63.5	64.0	64.5	65.0	65.5	66.0	66.5	67.0	67.5
47.5	19	19								
48.0	20	20	20	19						
48.5	21	21	20	20	20	19				
49.0	21	21	21	21	20	20	20	19	19	
49.5	22	22	22	21	21	21	20	20	20	19
50.0	23	23	22	22	22	21	21	21	21	20
50.5	24	23	23	23	23	22	22	22	21	21
51.0	25	24	24	24	23	23	23	22	22	22
51.5	25	25	25	24	24	24	23	23	23	22
52.0	26	26	25	25	25	24	24	24	23	23
52.5	27	26	26	26	25	25	25	24	24	24

53.0	27	27	27	26	26	26	25	25	25	24
53.5	28	28	27	27	27	26	26	26	25	25
54.0	29	28	28	28	27	27	27	26	26	26
54.5	29	29	29	28	28	28	27	27	27	26
55.0	30	30	29	29	29	28	28	28	27	27
55.5	31	30	30	30	29	29	29	28	28	28
56.0	31	31	30	30	30	30	29	29	29	28
56.5	32	31	31	31	30	30	30	29	29	29
57.0	32	32	32	31	31	31	30	30	30	29
57.5	33	33	32	32	32	31	31	31	30	30
58.0	34	33	33	33	32	32	32	31	31	31
58.5	34	34	34	33	33	33	32	32	32	31
59.0	35	35	34	34	34	33	33	33	32	32
59.5	35	35	35	34	34	34	33	33	33	33
60.0	36	36	35	35	35	34	34	34	33	33
60.5	37	36	36	36	35	35	35	34	34	34
61.0	37	37	37	36	36	36	35	35	35	34
61.5	38	37	37	37	36	36	36	36	35	35
62.0	38	38	38	37	37	37	36	36	36	35
62.5	39	39	38	38	38	37	37	37	36	36
63.0	40	39	39	39	38	38	38	37	37	37
63.5	40	40	39	39	39	38	38	38	37	37
64.0	41	40	40	40	39	39	39	38	38	38
64.5	41	41	41	40	40	40	39	39	39	38
65.0	42	41	41	41	40	40	40	39	39	39
65.5	42	42	42	41	41	41	40	40	40	39
66.0	43	42	42	42	41	41	41	41	40	40
66.5	43	43	43	42	42	42	41	41	41	40
67.0	44	44	43	43	43	42	42	42	41	41
67.5	44	44	44	43	43	43	42	42	42	41
68.0	45	45	44	44	44	43	43	43	42	42
68.5	45	45	45	44	44	44	43	43	43	43
69.0	46	46	45	45	45	44	44	44	43	43
69.5	46	46	46	45	45	45	44	44	44	44
70.0	47	47	46	46	46	45	45	45	44	44
70.5			47	46	46	46	46	45	45	45
71.0				47	47	46	46	46	45	45
71.5						47	47	46	46	46

275

72.0							47	47	46	46
72.5									47	47

PERCENT BODY FAT ESTIMATION FOR WOMEN (HEIGHT RANGE 5'8" to 6'½")

CIRCUMFERENCE VALUE	HEIGHT IN INCHES									
	68.0	68.5	69.0	69.5	70.0	70.5	71.0	71.5	72.0	72.5
49.5	19									
50.0	20	20	19							
50.5	21	20	20	20	19	19				
51.0	21	21	21	20	20	20	19	19		
51.5	22	22	21	21	21	20	20	20	20	19
52.0	23	22	22	22	21	21	21	21	20	20
52.5	23	23	23	22	22	22	22	21	21	21
53.0	24	24	23	23	23	22	22	22	22	21
53.5	25	24	24	24	23	23	23	23	22	22
54.0	25	25	25	24	24	24	24	23	23	23
54.5	26	26	25	25	25	24	24	24	24	23
55.0	27	26	26	26	25	25	25	25	24	24
55.5	27	27	27	26	26	26	25	25	25	25
56.0	28	28	27	27	27	26	26	26	25	25
56.5	29	28	28	28	27	27	27	26	26	26
57.0	29	29	29	28	28	28	27	27	27	26
57.5	30	29	29	29	29	28	28	28	27	27
58.0	30	30	30	29	29	29	29	28	28	28
58.5	31	31	30	30	30	29	29	29	29	28
59.0	32	31	31	31	30	30	30	29	29	29
59.5	32	32	32	31	31	31	30	30	30	29
60.0	33	32	32	32	32	31	31	31	30	30
60.5	33	33	33	32	32	32	32	31	31	31
61.0	34	34	33	33	33	32	32	32	32	31
61.5	35	34	34	34	33	33	33	32	32	32
62.0	35	35	35	34	34	34	33	33	33	32
62.5	36	35	35	35	34	34	34	34	33	33
63.0	36	36	36	35	35	35	34	34	34	34
63.5	37	37	36	36	36	35	35	35	34	34
64.0	37	37	37	36	36	36	36	35	35	35

64.5	38	38	37	37	37	36	36	36	36	35
65.0	38	38	38	38	37	37	37	36	36	36
65.5	39	39	38	38	38	37	37	37	37	36
66.0	40	39	39	39	38	38	38	37	37	37
66.5	40	40	39	39	39	39	38	38	38	37
67.0	41	40	40	40	39	39	39	39	38	38
67.5	41	41	41	40	40	40	39	39	39	38
68.0	42	41	41	41	40	40	40	40	39	39
68.5	42	42	42	41	41	41	40	40	40	39
69.0	43	42	42	42	41	41	41	41	40	40
69.5	43	43	43	42	42	42	41	41	41	41
70.0	44	43	43	43	43	42	42	42	41	41
70.5	44	44	44	43	43	43	42	42	42	42
71.0	45	44	44	44	44	43	43	43	42	42
71.5	45	45	45	44	44	44	43	43	43	42
72.0	46	45	45	45	45	44	44	44	43	43
72.5	46	46	46	45	45	45	44	44	44	44
73.0	47	46	46	46	45	45	45	45	44	44
73.5		47	47	46	46	46	45	45	45	44
74.0				47	46	46	46	46	45	45
74.5					47	47	46	46	46	45
75.0							47	46	46	46
75.5								47	47	46
76.0										47

APPENDIX B

A Sample Four-Week

Lean Look

Meal Plan

The following four-week meal plan is based on the key food substitution and "substitute staple" foods presented in chapter 5 and can provide guidance for your eating choices in Phase I. (Note that the meal plan does not fully integrate the nutrient timing strategies that are introduced in Phase II, but by now you should know how to incorporate the techniques on your own using the meals and snacks suggested here.)

WEEK 1

	Day 1	Day 2	Day 3	Day 4	Day 5	Day 6	Day 7
Break-fast	Whole-wheat pancakes Reduced-fat yogurt with diced fruit	Reduced-fat yogurt with frozen berries Bran muffin	Oatmeal with 1% milk and banana Cottage cheese	100 percent whole-wheat, rye or multigrain toast Scrambled egg whites with vegetable salsa	Low-fat apple cinnamon muffin Peanut butter Orange	100 percent bran ceral with 1 percent milk/soy milk and raisins	Whole-wheat English muffin Scrambled egg with melted cheese Turkey bacon 1/2 grapefruit
Lunch	Mixed salad greens Chicken fajitas Apple	Cheese Pizza with whole-wheat crust Raw veggies with low-fat ranch dressing	Minestrone soup Open-faced tuna melt Grapes	Whole-wheat wrap with turkey breast/ Black Forest ham/Lean roast beef with spinach, avocado green/red peppers Pineapple	Fresh fruit salad with 1 percent cottage cheese mixed with reduced-fat yogurt Whole-wheat roll	Vegetable beef soup Egg salad sandwich Carrot and celery sticks	PB&J on whole-wheat bread Orange juice
Dinner	Whole-wheat pasta with tomato meat sauce Vegetable salad with low-fat dressing	Sweet 'n sour chicken stir-fry with red peppers, broccoli, onions, mushroom, and pineapple	Grilled salmon Baked potato with light sour cream Garden salad with light dressing Steamed veggies (e.g., green beans or peas)	Grilled skinless chicken breast with low-fat Fettuccine Alfredo Asparagus or peas Low-fat coleslaw	Lean cut pork loin chop or pork tenderloin Brown/wild rice Steamed green beans Raw veggies and reduced-fat dip	Homemade burgers (95 percent lean meat) with whole-wheat bun Spinach salad with reduced-fat dressing	Whole-wheat soft tacos with meat, shredded lettuce, tomatoes, and cheddar Spanish rice Shredded carrot and raisin salad
Snacks for the day	Apple Light Cheddar cheese Whole-wheat toast	Yogurt Nuts Grapes	1 percent milk Low-fat cookies (e.g., gingersnaps, graham wafer crackers, etc.) Orange	Applesauce Trail mix Low-fat granola bar	Light Cheddar cheese Cantaloupe Frozen yogurt	Raw veggies with reduced-fat dip Fruit salad with yogurt or cottage cheese	Peanut Butter and whole-wheat crackers Banana

WEEK 2

	Day 1	Day 2	Day 3	Day 4	Day 5	Day 6	Day 7
Break-fast	Multigrain English muffin with 2 egg whites, 1 slice cheese	Whole-grain cereal, with raisins, sliced banana, 1 percent milk	Whole-wheat pancakes with fresh blueberries Scrambled egg whites	Low-fat bran muffin Low-fat cheese 1/2 grapefruit	Egg white omelet with veggies and salsa Whole-grain toast	Cottage cheese and fruit salad Multigrain toast	Whole-grain bagel with natural peanut butter or light cream cheese Strawberries
Lunch	Whole-wheat wrap with Black Forest ham, cheese, spinach and red peppers Yogurt and fruit	Pasta salad: whole-wheat rotini noodles with carrots, broccoli, cauliflower, onions, black olives tossed with light Italian dressing; add barbecued chicken or cottage cheese	Leftover tacos: ground meat, whole-wheat soft tortillas, chopped tomatoes, shredded lettuce and cheese; rice and salsa	Mac and cheese: Whole-wheat macaroni noodles, canned tuna (drained), green peppers, grated Cheddar	Veggie pizza Orange juice Yogurt and fruit	Roast beef in a whole-wheat bun Spinach salad with strawberries and toasted almonds	Scrambled eggs with salsa Whole-grain rye toast Raw veggies with low-fat ranch dressing
Supper	Grilled salmon Whole-wheat couscous Broccoli sprinkled with Parmesan cheese	Tacos: ground meat (buffalo or turkey), whole-wheat soft tortillas, chopped tomatoes, shredded lettuce and cheese; rice and salsa	Grilled Salmon Steamed brown rice Corn on the cob	BBQ skinless chicken breast Steamed grean beans	Chicken quesadillas: barbecued chicken, green chiles, Monterey Jack cheese, whole-wheat tortillas Salad	Chicken stir-fry with brown rice, frozen peas, chopped onion, and dash of soy sauce Salad	Whole-wheat spaghettini noodles with lean meat sauce Multigrain dinner roll Vegetable salad
Snacks for the day	Low-fat cheese Low-sodium Wheat Thins Sliced apples	Low-fat yogurt Fresh berries Low-fat granola	Antipasto and whole-wheat crackers Snack mix: nuts, raisins, Multigrain Cheerios	Low-fat granola Grapes Almonds	Cottage cheese and/or yogurt with sliced fruit Peanut butter on graham wafer crackers	1/2 grapefruit NutriGrain bar or Fruit Source bar Low-fat milk pudding	Smoothie: milk, yogurt, fruit, ice Fig Newton cookies

WEEK 3

	Day 1	Day 2	Day 3	Day 4	Day 5	Day 6	Day 7
Break-fast	Breakfast burrito: whole-wheat wrap with scrambled eggs, cheese, salsa, green pepper, onion, mushrooms	Whole-grain Cheerios or All-Bran cereal 1 percent milk Fruit salad	Multigrain bagel with peanut butter, banana 100 percent fruit juice	Breakfast sandwich: whole-wheat English muffin with eggs, cheese, and tomato Orange juice	Oatmeal with 1 percent milk, dried cranberries	Whole-wheat frozen waffles with strawberries and cottage cheese	Smoothie: frozen berries, yogurt, 1 percent milk, banana Whole-grain toast
Lunch	Turkey sandwich: whole-grain bread with turkey, sliced tomato, peppers, lettuce, and mustard Applesauce	Leftover spaghetti and meat sauce Sliced cucumbers Yogurt	Chef salad: leaf lettuce with grated cheese, sliced turkey, ham, reduced-fat dressing Whole-grain bun	Vegetable beef soup Egg salad sandwich Carrot and celery sticks	Veggie pizza V8 juice Cantaloupe or melon	Leftover Hamburger Helper wrapped in tortilla Raw carrots Yogurt	Spread peanut butter over pita bread and wrap around a banana Skim milk Cherry tomatoes
Supper	Spaghetti with turkey meat sauce Tossed salad with light vinaigrette Frozen yogurt	BBQ skinless chicken breast on whole-wheat bun Salad with sugar snap peas, bean sprouts, vinaigrette Strawberries	Black bean tortilla soup Glass of 1 percent milk Grape tomatoes	Baked fish Brown basmati rice Steamed broccoli and cauliflower Canned fruit	Hamburger Helper with buffalo meat Romaine lettuce salad with reduced-fat dressing	Pork stir-fry: noodles with stir-fry sauce, frozen mixed Asian vegetables, sliced pork loin or sliced pork tenderloin Fresh fruit	Homemade pizza: whole-wheat pizza crust, tomato sauce, green peppers, mushrooms, tomato, grated cheese
Snacks for the day	Cottage cheese with sliced pear Granola bar	Skim chocolate milk Kiwis	Yogurt Muesli Sliced apple	Low-fat oatmeal cookies 1 percent milk Piece of fruit	Yogurt and canned fruit Raw veggies and light dip	Low-fat granola Almonds 1 percent milk	Dried fruit Raw veggies and dip

WEEK 4

	Day 1	Day 2	Day 3	Day 4	Day 5	Day 6	Day 7
Break-fast	French toast with diced strawberries Turkey bacon	Oatmeal Toast and natural peanut butter 1 percent milk	Whole-grain English muffin with poached egg, slice or cheese, and salsa	Flavored oatmeal with cottage cheese, sliced fruit, 1 percent milk	Scrambled or poached egg on whole-grain rye bread Sliced tomato	100 percent bran cereal with 1 percent milk, Cran-Raisins	Whole-wheat pancakes Turkey bacon Mixed berries 1 percent milk
Lunch	Barbecued skinless chicken breast Cottage cheese	Whole-wheat pita stuffed with oven-roasted turkey or roast beef, green peppers, sprouts, and tomatoes	Tuna casserole: cooked whole-wheat macaroni, canned tuna, peppers and olives tossed with grated mozzarella cheese	Minestrone soup low-fat cheese and crackers Apple	Whole-wheat wrap with pastrami, grated carrots, shredded lettuce, sliced cucumber Fruit	Marinated chicken on skewers Vegetable salad Baked potato with salsa	Soft-shell tacos with ground buffalo or turkey, tomatoes, shredded lettuce, salsa, grated cheese
Supper	Whole-wheat spaghetti with tomato and turkey meat sauce Raw vegetable pieces with low-fat dressing	Thai chicken stir-fry with bean sprouts, broccoli, green onions, mushrooms, celery, snow peas Steamed brown rice	Homemade lean hamburger patties Oven-roasted sweet potato wedges tossed with olive oil and nutmeg or rosemary Steamed asparagus	Grilled salmon or sole Whole-wheat macaroni tossed with olive oil and mushrooms Shredded carrot and raisin salad	Pork loin chop or pork tenderloin Wild rice with lemon and herbs Steamed green beans Veggies and low-fat dip	Sweet 'n sour meatballs with red peppers and pineapple Steamed brown rice Spinach salad with reduced-fat dressing	Pasta salad: whole-wheat rotini noodles, chicken breast or cottage cheese, broccoli, carrots, celery, onions, tossed with light Italian dressing
Snacks for the day	Low-fat yogurt Low-fat granola Blueberries	Low-sodium Wheat Thin crackers with natural peanut butter Pear	Sesame snaps Orange Low-fat granola with cran-raisins	Low-fat yogurt Trail mix Strawberries	Fruit salad with yogurt or cottage cheese Graham crackers	Raw veggies with reduced-fat dip Air-popped popcorn	V8 vegetable juice Banana Pretzels

APPENDIX C

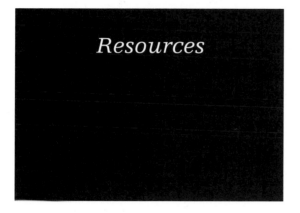

Resources

Various types of exercise equipment, gear, and other products have been mentioned and discussed in this book. Below is information that will help you shop for any such items you might be interested in purchasing.

BODY FAT SCALES

Popular Brands
HoMedics
Ironman (by Tanita)
Jenny Craig (by Tanita)
Oregon Scientific

Where to Buy

Amazon.com
Body Trends (www.bodytrends.com)
CVS Pharmacy

Phoenix

Tanita

Taylor

Weight Watchers (by Tanita)

Drugstore.com

REI

Sport Chalet

Target (www.target.com), Walgreens

Wal-Mart (www.walmart.com)

CABLE RESISTANCE

Popular Brands

Altus Athletic Home/
Door Gym

Everlast Pilates Door Gym
(with adjustable tension)

Lifeline Off-The-Wall Gym

Life Fitness G5

Where to Buy

AmericanFitness.net

Cannon Sports

Dick's Sporting Goods

Drugstore.com

Dunham's Sports, Lifefitness.com

Olympia Sports

Sport Chalet

The Sports Authority

EXERCISE BENCHES

Popular Brands

Body-Solid

Marcy

Nautilus

ProForm

Weider

Where to Buy

Bigfitness.com

Dick's Sporting Goods

Play It Again Sports

Sears (www.sears.com)

Busy Body Home Fitness

The Sports Authority

Wal-Mart (www.walmart.com)

SELECTORIZED DUMBBELLS

Popular Brands

Bowflex SelectTech

PowerBlock

ProBell

Where to Buy

2nd Wind Exercise

Bigfitness.com

Busy Body Home Fitness

Bowflexselecttech.com

Dick's Sporting Goods

Dunham's Sports

Gym Source

OMNI Fitness Equipment

Play It Again Sports

Powerblock.com

Probell.com

Sears (www.sears.com)

The Sports Authority

STABILITY BALLS

Popular Brands

Duraball

Resist-A-Ball

SPRI Xercise Ball

Stamina

Where to Buy

Dick's Sporting Goods

Sport Chalet

Target (www.target.com)

The Sports Authority

Walgreens

Wal-Mart (www.walmart.com)

Performbetter.com

BICYCLES

Popular Brands	Where to Buy
Cannondale	Cannondale.com
Schwinn	Performance Bicycle
Specialized	REI
Trek	Schwinn.com
	Specialized.com
	Trekbikes.com

STATIONARY BIKES

Popular Brands	Where to Buy
Life Fitness	Dick's Sporting Goods
NordicTrack	Play It Again Sports
Precor	Sears (www.sears.com)
ProForm	Target (www.target.com)
Reebok	The Sports Authority
Schwinn	

ELLIPTICAL TRAINERS AND STAIR CLIMBERS

Popular Brands	Where to Buy
Life Fitness	Busy Body
NordicTrack	Dick's Sporting Goods
Precor	Play It Again Sports
ProForm	Sears (www.sears.com)
Reebok	Target (www.target.com)
Schwinn	The Sports Authority

SLIDE BOARDS

Popular Brands

Exerslide

Goaler One

Professional

ULTRASLIDE

Where to Buy

Amazon.com

Betterhockey.com

Lifestylesport.com

Jumpusa.com

Performbetter.com

HEART RATE MONITORS

Popular Brands

Cardiosport

Garmin

Nike

Polar

Reebok

Timex Ironman

Where to Buy

Bodytronics.com

Dick's Sporting Goods

Performance Bike

REI

Sport Chalet

The Sports Authority

INLINE SKATES

Popular Brands

Bauer

K2

Roces

Rollerblade

Where to Buy

Dick's Sporting Goods

Sport Chalet

Target (www.target.com)

The Sports Authority

INDEX

abdominal muscles. *See* core exercises
accuracy, tape measure method and, 18
Achilles tendon stretches, 194
adaptive momentum, resistance exercise
    and, 24
advanced level
    Phase I workout schedules, 36, 96–97,
        118
    Phase II workout schedules, 124–25,
        181–84, 190
    Phase III workout schedules, 201,
        241–44, 241–44, 250
    suggested workouts, 93, 176, 236
aerobic exercise. *See* cardio exercise
age, body fat percentages and, 12, 13
alcoholic beverages, 48
alternating shoulder presses, 167
appetite, weight and, 38–39

appetizers, nutrient timing and, 129, 135–37
Armstrong, Lance, 245
athletes
    body fat percentages and, 3–4, 16, 17
    circuit workouts and, 23, 24
Atkins Diet, 9
attractiveness, leanness and, 8–9

back pain, 23, 191
back stretches, 192
beginner level
    Phase I workout schedule, 36, 94–95,
        117
    Phase II workout schedules, 123–24,
        177–80, 189
    Phase III workout schedules, 199–200,
        237–40, 249
    suggested workouts, 92, 175, 235

bent-over cable rowing, 160
bent-over cable side shoulder raises, 172
beta-alanine, 204–6, 215
beverages, 40, 45–48, 129, 140–42
biceps and front shoulder stretches, 191
biceps curls, 169
bicycling, 99–101
bioelectrical impedance, 15
bitter orange, 216
Bod Pods, 2, 14
body fat percentages
    dieting and, 11
    healthy ranges for, 12–13
    measuring, 14–19, 121, 267–77
    weight and, 2, 4, 7, 8
body fat scales, 12, 15–16
bone density, resistance exercise and, 23
boredom, avoiding, 258–59
breads, 53
breakfast, 129, 130–31, 132
"bulking up," fear of, 146–47
buttocks stretches, 193–94

cable curls and presses, 170
cable front shoulder raises, 88
cable pull-downs, 75
cable resistance devices, 63, 222
cable side shoulder raises, 87
caffeine, 216
caffeine drinks, 46–47
calf stretches, 194
calories
    burning, 22–23, 25, 146, 256
    calorically dense foods, 39, 41–42
    counting, 40–41
    food substitutions and, 57
    low-calorie diets, 9–10
    nutrient timing and, 127–28
carbohydrates, 134, 135, 138, 140, 141
cardiac lag, 254–55
cardio exercise
    avoiding injuries and, 188–94
    bicycling, 99–101
    elliptical training and stair climbing,
        101–3

foundation workouts and, 260
heart rate monitoring and, 250–57
inline skating, 103–5
Lean Look Program overview and, 4–5,
        25–27
mixed intervals workout, 261
Phase I and, 33–34, 109–16
Phase II and, 123
Phase III and, 197, 199, 245–57
running, 105–6
swimming, 106–8
tempo workouts, 260–61
walking, 108–9
workout schedules, 117–18
cardiovascular disease, 10–11
CCK (satiety peptide), 136, 137
cereals, 53
chest dips, 165
chest stretches, 191
chin-ups, 159
chitosan, 217
chocolate, dark, 55
cholesterol, 8
chondroitin, 210, 215
chromium, 217
circuit workouts, 22, 23–24
circulating inflammation markers, 8
Complete Book of Food Counts, The (Netzer),
        57
core exercises, 65, 74–81, 157–64, 227–29
creatine, 206–7, 215
crunch twists, 162

dairy foods, 40, 54
desserts, 40, 45, 55–56
diabetes, 141
dietary supplements. See nutritional
        supplements
dieting, 5, 9–11, 20, 57
diet pills, 216–18
diet sodas, 47
disease risks, 2, 8, 25–26, 206, 207
dogs, walking, 259, 260
Dolan, Mike, 2
double-leg bucks, 73

dumbbell flye exercises, 82
dumbbell rows, 74
dumbbells, 62, 222

eating out, food substitutions and, 40
eating slowly, nutrient timing and, 138–39
eggs, 50
elderly people, muscle mass and, 8
electrode jels, 253
elliptical training and stair climbing, 101–3
energy balance, 10
energy needs, nutrient timing and, 127–29,
        130, 133–34
equipment
        avoiding injuries and, 189–90
        cardio exercise and, 99–104, 106, 107,
                108–9
        heart rate monitors, 251–56
        resistance exercise and, 25, 61, 62–63,
                90, 91, 148
        sources of, 283–87
excess postexercise oxygen consumption
        (OPEC), 234
exercise benches, 62–63
exercise logs, 256

failure
        dieting and, 20
        lifestyle changes and, 22
fall workout schedule, 260, 265
fast repetitions, power development and,
        219–20
fat, losing, 7, 23, 25, 26
fat mass. *See* body fat percentages
feedback information, heart rate monitoring
        and, 256, 257
fiber, 41, 44, 52, 207–8, 215
fish, 48, 49, 50
fish oil, 209, 215
flaxseed oil, 209, 215
food choices. *See* nutrition
food substitutions, 5, 21, 22, 33–34, 38–41,
        57–58, 266
        beverages, 45–48
        dairy foods, 54

desserts, 55–56
fried foods, 48–49
fruits, 44–45
meats, 49–50
nutritional supplements, 203–4
organic foods, 56–57
sauces and condiments, 51–52
vegetables, 41–44
whole grains, 52–53
forward lunges, 152
foundation workouts, cardio exercise and,
        260
4-minute intervals, 246, 247
freestyle swimming, 107
fried foods, 40, 48–49
fruits, 39, 42, 44–45, 55

garcinia, 217
gelatin-based desserts, 55
gender, body fat percentages and,
        12, 13
GLP-1 (satiety peptide), 136
glucosomine, 210, 215
glycemic index (GI), 138
goals, body fat percentages and, 13
good morning exercises, 79
grains, whole, 52–53
groin stretches, 193

hamstrings stretches, 193
health
        body fat percentages and, 2, 12–13
        disease risks, 2, 8, 25–26, 206, 207
        fiber and, 208
        resistance exercise and, 23
        vitamins and minerals, 211–12
        weight and, 8
heart disease. *See* cardiovascular disease
heart rate monitoring, 250–57, 259–60
heart rate zones, 253–54
heel dips, 72
heel raises, 70
hip flexors stretches, 192
hoodia gordonii, 217
hunger, low-calorie diets, 10

hydration, 16
hypertrophy, 23

iliotibial band stretches, 193
incline power push-ups, 231
injuries, 23, 104–5, 188–94
inline skating, 103–5
insulin, nutrient timing and, 124, 133, 135
intermediate intervals, 185–88, 189, 190, 246
interval workouts
    cardio exercise and, 26, 109–16
    mixed intervals workout, 261
    Phase I and, 109–18
    Phase II and, 123, 185–88, 189
    Phase III and, 199, 245–50
    swimming and, 108

Jensen, Karen, 3
joint pain, 210

Lean Look Program
    cardio exercise and, 25–27
    maintaining, 258–66
    nutrition and, 21–22
    overview, 20–21
    readiness and, 29–30
    resistance exercise and, 22–25
    workout schedules, 27–29, 262–65
leanness, 3–4, 7–11
leg exercises, 67–73, 149–56, 224–26
long intervals, 199, 245–50
L-overs, 161
low-calorie diets, 9–10, 11
low-density lipoprotein (LDL) cholesterol, 8
low-fat foods, 55–56
lying hip adductions, 68

maintaining the Lean Look program, 258–66
meal plans, 278–82
measurements, body fat percentages, 11–12, 14–19
meats, 40, 49–50, 56

memory features, heart rate monitoring and, 256
men, body fat percentages and, 16, 17, 268–72
military, U.S., body fat percentages and, 16
minerals. See vitamins and minerals
mixed intervals workout, 261
mortality rates, weight cycling and, 10–11
mountain climber exercises, 229
multi-joint exercises, 24
muscle balancing exercises
    avoiding injuries and, 190–91
    Phase I and, 24, 34, 59–61, 90–93
    Phase II and, 147–48
    Phase III and, 221–22
muscle groups, 90, 91, 148
muscle mass, 8, 11, 23, 214–15
muscle strength, 7, 59–61, 146, 205, 206
muscular endurance workouts, 261

Netzer, Corinne T., 57
normal weight obesity, 2, 8, 17
nutrient timing, 21, 22, 41, 122, 266
    appetizers and, 129, 135–37
    breakfast and, 129, 130–31
    energy needs and, 127–29
    overeating, avoiding and, 129, 138–39
    snacks and, 129, 131–33, 139–40
    sports drinks and, 129
    workout schedules and, 129, 133–35, 137–38, 142–44
nutrition, 4, 5, 21–22, 266
    food substitutions and, 33–34, 38–57
    nutrient timing and, 122, 126–44
    nutritional supplements and, 197, 198, 202–18
nutritional supplements, 21–22, 202–4, 266
    beta-alanine, 204–6, 215
    creatine, 206–7, 215
    diet pills, 216–18
    fiber, 207–8, 215
    fish oil and flaxseed oil, 209, 215
    glucosomine and chondroitin, 210, 215
    vitamins and minerals, 211–13, 215
    whey protein, 213–15, 216

oblique crunches, 77
olive oil, 48
omega-3 fatty acids, 209
1-minute interval workouts, 34, 110–11, 112, 115–16, 185
one-arm dumbbell snatches, 230
organic foods, 40, 56–57, 202
overeating, avoiding, 129, 131, 138–39
overuse injuries. *See* injuries
overworking, heart rate monitoring and, 255
oxygen deficits, 234

Parathesia, 206
pedometers, 259
periodization, 24, 246, 258–59
Phase I
 cardio exercise, 26, 33–34, 98–118
 nutrition, 33–34
 resistance exercise, 33, 59–97
 workout schedules, 34, 94–97
Phase II
 cardio exercise, 26, 121, 123, 185–94
 nutrition, 121, 122, 126–44
 resistance exercise, 121, 122, 145–84
 workout schedules, 123–25
Phase III
 cardio exercise, 26–27, 197, 199
 nutrition, 197, 198, 202–18
 resistance exercise, 197, 198, 219–43
 workout schedules, 199–201, 249–50
"plus-five rule," 260–61
"plus-one rule"
 cardio exercise, 186, 246, 260–61
 heart rate monitoring and, 254
 resistance exercise, 61, 65–66, 147, 223, 261
power development exercises, 24, 198, 219–44
power interval workouts
 Phase I, 34, 112, 114–15
 Phase II and, 185
preparations, Phase I, 61–66
pre-workout meals, 129, 137–38
processed foods, 39

protein, 129, 134, 135, 139–40, 141–42, 213–15
push-ups, 85
PYY (satiety peptide), 136

quadriceps stretches, 192

readiness, Lean Look Program and, 29–30
recovery nutrition, 129, 133–35
resistance exercise
 core exercises, 74–81, 157–64, 227–29
 Lean Look Program and, 4–5, 22–25
 leg exercises, 67–73, 149–56, 224–26
 Phase I, 33, 59–97
 Phase II, 122, 145–84
 Phase III, 197, 198, 219–43
 preparations for, 61–66
 upper body exercises, 82–89, 165–72, 230–32
 workout schedules, 94–97, 177–84, 237–44
reverse crunches, 163
reverse wood chop exercises, 232
Romanian deadlifts, 67
rotator cuff stretches, 191–92
running, 105–6

salads, 42
satiety, nutrient timing and, 135–36
saturated fats, 54
sauces and condiments, 40, 51–52
scissor jumps, 224
"setting your core," resistance exercise and, 61, 65
7-Keto, 217
short intervals, 109–18, 254–55
shoulder presses, 83
shoulder shrugs, 84
side plank exercises, 80
side shoulder raises, 86
side step-ups, 71
Singh, Devendra, 9
single-leg box jumps, 225
single-leg squats with stability ball, 150
6-minute intervals, 247–48

skinniness, 7–8
slide boards, 103
snacks, 45, 129, 131–33, 137, 139–40
soda, 46, 47
South Beach diet, 9
speed interval workouts, 34, 112–13, 185
split squats, 153
sports drinks, 129, 140–42
spring workout schedule, 260, 263
squats with dumbbells, 151
stability ball back extensions, 164
stability ball crunches, 81
stability ball leg curls, 154
stability balls, 63
stability ball triceps presses, 168
stair climbers, 102–3
standing one-arm cable pulldowns, 228
standing single-arm cable flyes, 166
standing single-leg squats, 69
stick crunches, 76
strength building exercises, 122, 145–48,
        221–22, 261
    core exercises, 157–64
    leg exercises, 149–56
    upper body exercises, 165–72
    workout schedules, 173–76, 177–84
stretches, avoiding injuries and, 191–94
substitutions, food choices and. See food
        substitutions
summer workout schedule, 260, 264
Sumo squats, 147, 149
superman exercises, 78
supine bridge heel raises, 156
supplements. See nutritional supplements
swimming, 106–8

tape measure method, 12, 15, 16–18,
        267–77
tempo workouts, 260–61
thermic effect of food (TEF), 130
3-minute interval workouts, 185, 187–88
time requirements. See also workout
        schedules
    cardio exercise and, 112, 113, 114–16,
        186

Lean Look Program and, 20, 259
    resistance exercise and, 25
treadmills, 106
triceps presses, 171
tuck jumps, 227
2-minute interval workouts, 185, 187

upper body exercises, 82–89, 165–72,
        230–32
upright cable row, 89

variation, workouts and, 26, 59–60, 190
vegetables, 39, 41–44
vitamins and minerals, 211–13, 215
V-ups, 157

waist circumference measurements, 19
walking, 106, 108–9, 259, 260
wall jumps, 226
wall squats, 68
warm-ups, 61, 64, 112, 148, 186
weekly measurements, 18–19
weight, 1–2, 4, 5, 7–8
weight cycling, 10–11
weighted heel raises, 155
weighted stability ball crunches, 158
weightlifting, 2–3
Weight Watchers, 9
whey protein, 213–15, 216
whole grains, 40, 52–53
winter workout schedule, 260, 262
women, 16, 17, 18, 146–47, 273–77
workouts, suggested, 92–93, 173–76, 233–36
workout schedules. See also interval
        workouts
    Lean Look Program overview, 27–29
    maintaining the Lean Look program
        and, 260, 262–65
    nutrient timing and, 129, 133–35,
        137–38, 142–44
    Phase I, 34, 36–37, 94–97
    Phase II, 123–25, 177–84, 189, 190
    Phase III, 199–201, 237–44, 249–50

yo-yo dieting, 10–11